EMOTIONS
& Essential Oils

EMOTIONS
& Essential Oils

A Modern Resource for Healing
Emotional Reference Guide

Third Edition
Revised Fall 2014

Emotions & Essential Oils
A Modern Resource for Healing
Emotional Reference Guide
Third Edition

© 2014 Enlighten
All rights reserved.

Enlighten Alternative Healing, LLC

No part of this book may be reproduced or transmitted in any form, or by any means, electronic or mechanical, including photocopying, without written permission from Enlighten.
ISBN 978-0-9850133-9-4

Published by:
Enlighten Alternative Healing, LLC
PO Box 1444, American Fork, UT 84003
www.enlightenhealing.com/deo/

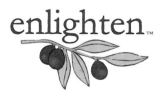

Notice to Readers:

The information contained in this book is for educational purposes only. It is not intended to diagnose, prescribe, or treat any emotional or physical condition, illness or injury. The author, publishers and distributors of this book shall have no liability or responsibility to any person or entity with respect to any and all alleged damage, loss or injury caused or alleged to be caused directly or indirectly by the information contained in this book. This book contains suggested uses of oils based on acceptable dosage amounts recommended by the manufacturer. The author makes no claim to have verified or validated these suggestions. The readers must validate acceptable dosage amounts from the manufacturer before application. The information in this book is in no way intended as a substitute for medical advice. Enlighten recommends that all readers obtain medical advice from a licensed health care professional before using essential oils for any reason.

"The medical school of the future will not particularly interest itself in the ultimate results and products of disease, nor will it pay so much attention to actual physical lesions, or administer drugs and chemicals merely for the sake of palliating our symptoms, but knowing the true cause of sickness and aware that the obvious physical results are merely secondary it will concentrate its efforts upon bringing about the harmony between body, mind and soul which results in the relief and cure of disease"

"Amongst the types of remedies that will be used will be those obtained from the most beautiful plants and herbs to be found in the pharmacy of Nature, such as have been divinely enriched with healing powers for the mind and body of man"

— *Dr. Edward Bach*

Table of Contents

Section I: Healing with Essential Oils

Kallie's Story 3
Healing Emotions with Essential Oils 7
A Word on Quality 11
How to Use Essential Oils 12
How to Use this Book 14
Citations 15

Section II: Oil Descriptions

Single Oils
  Arborvitae 20
  Basil 21
  Bergamot 22
  Birch 23
  Black Pepper 24
  Cardamom 25
  Cassia 26
  Cedarwood 27
  Cilantro 28
  Cinnamon 29
  Clary Sage 30
  Clove 31
  Coriander 32
  Cypress 33
  Eucalyptus 34
  Fennel 35

Frankincense 36
Geranium 37
Ginger 38
Grapefruit 39
Helichrysum 40
Jasmine 41
Juniper Berry 42
Lavender 43
Lemon 44
Lemongrass 45
Lime 46
Marjoram 47
Melaleuca 48
Melissa 49
Myrrh 50
Oregano 51
Patchouli 52
Peppermint 53
Roman Chamomile 54
Rose 55
Rosemary 56
Sandalwood 57
Tangerine 58
Thyme 59
Vetiver 60
White Fir 61
Wild Orange 62
Wintergreen 63
Ylang Ylang 64

Oil Blends
Introducing Oil Blends **66**
    Anti-Aging Blend 67
    Calming Blend 68
    Cleansing Blend 69
    Detoxification Blend 70
    Digestive Blend 71
    DNA Repairing Blend 72
    Focus Blend 73
    Grounding Blend 74
    Invigorating Blend 75
    Joyful Blend 76
    Massage Blend 77
    Metabolic Blend 78
    Monthly Blend 79
    Protective Blend 80
    Repellent Blend 81
    Respiratory Blend 82
    Skin Clearing Blend 83
    Soothing Blend 84
    Tension Blend 85
    Women's Blend 86

Section III: Appendices

Appendix A: Suggested Uses 91
Appendix B: Choosing and Applying Oils
    with Energy/Muscle Testing 114
Appendix C: Essential Oil Emotional Usage Guide 120
Appendix D: How to Host a Class 143
How to Order Books 149

Section I

Healing with Essential Oils

Kallie's Story

The following true story, written by Kallie's mother, perfectly embodies the steps involved in emotional healing—from the time of trauma, through the healing crisis and on to wholeness. It beautifully illustrates how the use of essential oils facilitates healing physically, emotionally and spiritually. We sincerely thank Kallie and her family for allowing this story to be included in this book.

When my daughter Kallie was two years old, she accidentally pulled a crock-pot full of boiling meat down onto herself, severely burning her face and torso. Second and third degree burns covered a third of her body. For a month Kallie recuperated in a special burn unit where she received heavy narcotics along with other medications to help numb the intense pain that accompanies such severe burns. Two surgeries were necessary to place skin grafts on her face, neck and shoulders. When Kallie finally came home, she had to wear a plastic mask on her face and a tight fitting body suit for six months to keep the skin grafts from warping.

As her mother, it was horrifying to see my child suffer so much pain. I felt helpless. But Kallie was a very strong girl who tried her best to adapt to the excruciating medical procedures, such as having the dead skin scrubbed from the burned area or working through physical therapy. During the many times when the pain and trauma were too much for little Kallie, she would mentally leave us. I could see it in her hollow eyes. The first time I saw this was when the initial burn happened. In those few seconds right after the hot liquid touched her precious skin, she wasn't there. Due to the combination of heavy narcotics and unbearable procedures, she was physically and emotionally numb or just plain absent during most of the month that she was hospitalized. After we got home, it took a while to get back to regular life.

Kallie was just so fragile and delicate. I tried my absolute best to physically and emotionally recover her and our family from this event, but it was quite a challenge.

The months and years went by and I started to notice that Kallie was extremely numb to pain. She was a very active, adventurous girl and would have quite a few falls and injuries just like any other child, but she would rarely acknowledge that it hurt her. Sometimes it was disturbing. I remember one visit to the doctor for her regular vaccines. Kallie was lying down on the table and the two nurses poked both her legs two times each. I was watching her face and there was absolutely no physical or emotional reaction whatsoever. She was unfeeling. She would often get nasty gashes or scrapes and I wouldn't even know about it until later when I would give her a bath or change her clothes. I would ask her where she got hurt and a lot of times she wouldn't even remember. She was also very self-conscious of the physical changes the burn had caused. When Kallie began school, she would try to hide her scars by covering them with her hair or coat or by walking with her face pointed towards the wall and away from onlookers.

I never pushed her to talk about it or do anything that was uncomfortable for her, but I gently tried to give her opportunities to share her thoughts and feelings. When Kallie was about five and a half, she started to forget what happened. She knew that something big occurred a long time ago, but she couldn't remember the details. Sometimes there was a trigger that sparked her memory, like the word "burn," or a fire, or even a bath. Then with fear and confusion in her eyes she would start asking, "What happened to me, Mom?" Around this time, I was introduced to essential oils. As my mother and I learned about the oils and their benefits, we thought of Kallie. Helichrysum and Vetiver seemed like the perfect fit and we began treatment. I was so excited in the beginning, mostly thinking of the potential physical healing and largely unaware of the emotional benefits.

Kallie was full of faith. She immediately said, "I know it's gonna make my burn melt away Mom!" I had no idea what was coming.

After only a few days of using the oils, Kallie started to act differently. The first thing I noticed was that she started to complain of physical pain for which we could find no reasonable explanation. Every time she would get the smallest cut or bruise, she would have major anxiety about it—very opposite from her recent tough and "numb-to-pain" reactions. She would cry for hours about a tiny cut or sliver and would say through tears, "Is it ever gonna go away?" Kallie spent a large portion of the day worrying about the smallest things. It was almost impossible to convince her to take a bath. She became extremely picky about the clothes she wore. If clothing touched her "wrong" or was at all tight, she wouldn't wear it. Any mention of her being burned or even the word "burn" would cause extreme fear. Anxiety attacks surfaced. Sometimes she would randomly sit on my lap and just cry. I would cry too.

I finally realized Kallie was going through a healing crisis brought on by the oils. It made perfect sense. Every odd thing that she was doing directly correlated to the burn or to her experience in the hospital. With the help of essential oils, her body was expelling or ejecting all of the pain and hidden emotions that were buried for so long.

We guessed that the healing would probably last for the same amount of time she had stayed in the hospital. This was exactly right. It lasted a month. I tried my best to validate what she was feeling and to help her as much as I could during this time. I learned that if I missed a day of putting on her oils, it was a bad day for her and the rest of the household! So, I kept up with it and the results were phenomenal.

After this difficult month I began to notice that words which had previously triggered a negative reaction from Kallie did not seem to bother her. She had a totally new and positive perspective. I could see plain as day that she was no longer coming from a place of fear. Instead of being self-conscious or shy, she was secure, strong and confident—a totally different Kallie.

As her mom, I can see without a doubt that these essential oils gave her such a beautiful new outlook on herself and her past traumatic experience. On the morning of Kallie's seventh birthday, I was telling her about the day she was born and she said, "I don't remember that, Mom, but I do remember when I was burned." I carefully asked, "What do you feel when you remember it?" She replied in her bubbly, secure voice, "Let me spell it for you mom: OK!" Words cannot express how very grateful I am that my little Kallie could heal emotionally.

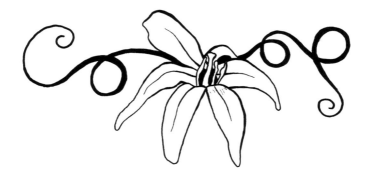

Healing Emotions
with Essential Oils

As was just illustrated in Kallie's story, essential oils play a powerful role in emotional healing. They lead us by the hand as we courageously face our emotional issues. Kallie is not the only one with repressed emotional trauma. We all hold unresolved feelings of pain and hurt which need to be brought to the surface for transformation and healing.

Essential Oils: Five Stages of Healing

Essential oils support healing in five stages. They strengthen us during each stage and prepare us for the next level of healing. For example, as we regain our physical health, we are invited to enter the emotional realm.

In this book we briefly explore stage one and mainly focus on defining stage two: the emotional stage. While we briefly touch on concepts from stages three through five in the oil descriptions, they are largely topics for another book.

The Five Stages are:

1. Essential oils assist in healing the physical body
2. Essential oils assist in healing the heart
3. Essential oils assist in releasing limiting beliefs
4. Essential oils increase spiritual awareness and connection
5. Essential oils inspire the fulfillment of our life's purpose

Stage One: Healing the Physical Body

Essential oils are powerful physical healers. Some essential oils are considered to be 40 to 60 times more potent than herbs. They have many "anti" qualities. The oils range from being anti-bacterial, to anti-viral and anti-parasitic in nature (Schnaubelt, 2011). Essential oils assist the body in fighting unfriendly micro-organisms; purifying organs, glands and body systems; balancing body functions and raising the body's vibration (Stewart, 2003).

Stage Two: Healing the Heart

As the oils secure our physical health, they provide us with the energy needed to penetrate the heart and enter the emotional realm. Essential oils raise the vibration of the physical body (Stewart, 2003). As the body lives in higher vibrations, lower energies (such as suppressed emotions) become unbearable. These feelings want to release. Stagnant anger, sadness, grief, judgment and low self-worth cannot exist in the environment of balance and peace which essential oils help to create.

Emotional healing occurs as old feelings surface and release (Moreton, 1992). Sometimes this experience is confused with regression. People may perceive they are going backwards or that the essential oils are not working. We are so used to symptomatic healing that we have been conditioned to view healing as the immediate cessation of all physical and emotional pain. In reality, the oils *are* working. They are working to permanently heal emotional issues by supporting individuals through their healing.

Principles of Healing: Release and Receive

It is important to understand that healing is a process. The process can be separated into two main principles: release and receive.

We must release trapped negative emotions before we can receive positive feelings. The old must go to make space for the new. We often want to skip this step, but it is a necessary one. We must be willing to experience the cleansing if we truly desire healing. Resisting the cleansing process makes healing more painful. We must surrender to the experience so that we may continue on the path of healing. The more we let go and trust, the more enjoyable this healing process can be.

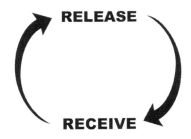

Essential Oils Don't Do Our Emotional Work for Us

Essential oils assist individuals in taking an honest look within. They foster the right environment for healing, but they will not do the work for us. In gardening, it is a common experience to pull the weeds while leaving the roots. This is particularly true for hard and rocky soils. To ensure we uproot the whole plant, we can add water to the soil, which allows the entire weed to be removed. Similarly, essential oils prepare our emotional soil so that weeds may be removed with greater ease. However, they do not do the weeding for us. If one neglects to do the work of pulling their weeds, they have simply watered the problem. On the other hand, those who combine essential oils with emotional work reap the fruit of their labor.

Tools for Emotional Work

You may be wondering, "How do I begin my emotional work?" We propose that individuals begin their emotional work with a few introductory practices. We suggest meditation, journaling and personal inventory to facilitate the healing process. We invite everyone to embark on their own healing path. We believe this book will greatly assist you and your family.

A Word on Quality

Three Categories of Essential Oils:

1. Aromatic Essential Oils
2. Therapeutic Grade Essential Oils
3. Independently Tested Therapeutic Grade Essential Oils

The first category applies to many oils marketed for their scent and aromatic properties. These essential oils are widely available in health food stores everywhere. It is important to know that these essential oils are not therapeutic grade and should not be used topically or internally, as they are not for medicinal use. These oils are usually synthetic and therefore harmful to the body. They have no therapeutic value whatsoever.

The second category of essential oils is therapeutic grade oils. Many companies fall into this category. The intent of these companies is to provide quality essential oils that can be used for healing. These oils are for topical and aromatic use. Great care should be taken when purchasing these oils, as they are often diluted with synthetic chemicals or other additives.

The third category of essential oils is independently tested therapeutic grade oils. These oils are tested at independent laboratories with tests such as gas chromatography and mass spectrometry to verify their purity and composition. Oils that meet rigorous testing and are considered safe by the Food and Drug Administration (FDA) may be considered for topical and internal use. Never use any essential oil internally that is not "generally recognized as safe" for dietary consumption by the FDA. Also consult with a health care professional. Only the highest quality essential oils should be used for physical, emotional and spiritual healing.

How to Use Essential Oils

Please take care to reference all safety information when using essential oils for aromatic, topical or internal use. (See "A Word on Quality" in this section.)

Aromatic

To use an essential oil aromatically, simply smell the oil directly from the bottle. You may also place a few drops into a diffuser which disperses the oil into the air. Another option is to place a few drops of the essential oil into the palms of the hands, rub together vigorously and inhale deeply.

Topical

To use an essential oil topically, place a few drops in the palm of the hand and apply to selected area(s). If you are using an essential oil that is irritating to the skin, dilute it with a carrier oil such as fractionated coconut oil. If you are applying more than one oil to the same place on your body, be sure to layer the oils rather than mixing them together first and applying them as a mixture. Layering means to apply the oils one at a time. Allow a few minutes for each oil to absorb into the skin before adding the next one. For suggestions on where to apply specific oils, see Appendix A.

Internal

Be sure to check all safety information from a competent reference book before ever using an essential oil internally. For more information on selecting quality oils see "A Word on Quality" in this section.

Caution: Use wisdom and consider all safety information from a competent reference book regarding essential oil use. There are some oils that should never be taken internally. Others should not be applied "neat," or directly on the skin, without first being diluted with a carrier oil. Also ensure the oils you are using are of the highest standards of quality. (See "A Word on Quality" in this section.) Use caution when using essential oils for children and babies. Some oils may not be safe for children or for use during pregnancy. Please read the instructions on the bottle, or check with the manufacturer to determine the safe uses of the oils. Essential oils can be much more potent than herbs, so a little goes a long way. Babies and children have highly sensitive skin and require less oil. If you are pregnant or nursing consult a licensed health care professional before applying essential oils.

How to Use This Book

Oil Descriptions

The main body of this book is divided into individual descriptions of the oils. The single oils are listed first and oil blends are next. You may read the individual or blend descriptions to determine which essential oil would be best suited for your emotional needs. You may then wish to reference the suggested uses in Appendix A and/or the information on applying oils through energy/muscle testing in Appendix B. If an essential oil doesn't seem to match your emotional state, but is similar, you may reference the companion oils listed at the bottom of the oil's description page to find a more applicable oil.

Usage Guide

In the Essential Oil Emotional Usage Guide (Appendix C) you may search for specific emotional states and find the recommended oil(s), which support those states.

Companion to Modern Essentials

This book may also be used as a companion to *Modern Essentials* (Modern Essentials, 2014), which serves as a reference guide to your physical health and application of essential oils. After finding the recommended oils for your physical condition, cross-reference those oils with the emotional descriptions found in this book. For the most powerful results, choose the oil(s) that match your emotional state as well as your physical condition.

Energy/Muscle Testing

If you are familiar with energy or muscle testing, you may reference information on applying oils through energy/muscle testing in Appendix B.

Citations

Moreton, V. S. (1992). A New Day in Healing!. (pp. 16-17). San Diego, CA: Kalos Publishing.

Schnaubelt, K. (2011). The Healing Intelligence of Essential Oils. (pp. 13-16). Rochester, Vermont: Healing Arts Press.

Stewart, D. (2003). Healing Oils of the Bible. (p. 31-34). Marble Hill, MO: Care Publications.

(2014). *Modern Essentials* . (Fifth Edition ed.). Spanish Fork: Aroma Tools. DOI: www.AromaTools.com

Section II

Oil Descriptions

SINGLE OILS

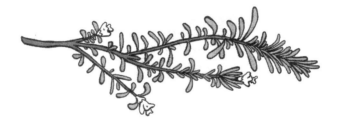

Arborvitae

The Oil of Divine Grace

Arborvitae assists individuals who believe or act like all progress must be made through struggle and solitary effort. Instead of trusting in the Divine, these individuals unconsciously block Divine aid, choosing instead to live by their own efforts. Arborvitae addresses the need to control one's outcomes in life. It invites individuals to live with peace and joy by trusting in the abundant flow of Divine grace.

Arborvitae is also a grounding oil which teaches that Divinity is all around us. God's grace can be felt and experienced here on earth; it is not distant or separate. God can help us find balance in our lives and know what we should hold close and what we should release.

Arborvitae's Latin name means "to sacrifice." This oil invites individuals to sacrifice their personal will and ambitions for a far more fulfilling way of living. By surrendering to God the mind relaxes and the soul experiences harmony and peace. Arborvitae teaches that true strength comes through emptiness or a willingness to receive God's strength. It asks individuals to relax, take a deep breath, and trust in the flow of life. Arborvitae assists the soul to live effortlessly by Divine grace.

Emotions Addressed: Willful, struggle, excessive effort, distrust, rigid, fearful, need to control

Companion Oils: Cypress, Sandalwood, Wintergreen, Massage Blend, Rose, Roman Chamomile

Basil

The Oil of Renewal

The symptoms of adrenal exhaustion help identify the main moods that are treated with Basil, primarily: overwhelm, fatigue, low energy and the inability to cope with life's stressors. The smell of Basil oil brings strength to the heart and relaxation to the mind. This oil is also excellent for states of nervousness, anxiety and depression.

Basil oil supports those who are under a great deal of mental strain. It brings rejuvenation of vital forces after long periods of burnout and exhaustion. Basil oil may strengthen the adrenals and restore the body to its natural rhythms of sleep, activity and rest.

Basil oil is also helpful for addiction recovery. It gives hope and optimism to the tired soul. Basil may assist an individual in giving up false stimulants or other substance related addictions. By increasing one's natural energy, it supports individuals to achieve greater balance and health. In short, Basil is indicated for those who are weary in mind and body and for those in need of strength and renewal.

Emotions Addressed: Anxious, weary, overwhelmed, tired, drained, exhausted, addicted

Companion Oils: Massage Blend, DNA Repairing Blend, Tension Blend

Bergamot

The Oil of Self-Acceptance

Bergamot relieves feelings of despair, self-judgment and low self-esteem. It supports the individual in need of self-acceptance and self-love. Bergamot invites individuals to see life with more optimism.

Bergamot has a cleansing affect on stagnant feelings and limiting belief systems. Because of individuals' core beliefs of being "bad," "unlovable" and "not good enough," they seek to hide behind a façade of cheerfulness. They may fear revealing their true thoughts and feelings. Bergamot's powerful cleansing properties generate movement in the energy system, which in turn brings hope.

In this way, Bergamot is a wonderful anti-depressant. It awakens the soul to hope and offers courage to share the inner-self. Re-igniting optimism and confidence in the Self, it imparts true self-acceptance. Bergamot teaches individuals to let go of self-judgment by learning to love themselves unconditionally.

Emotions Addressed: Despair, low self-esteem, self-judgment, unlovable, hopeless

Companion Oils: Metabolic Blend, Skin Clearing Blend, Cassia, Melissa

Birch

The Oil of Support

Birch offers support to the unsupported. When a person is feeling attacked or unsupported by family or friends, Birch offers courage to move forward alone. Learning to be flexible is important, but so is gaining a strong backbone. Birch offers support to the weak-willed to stand tall and firm in what they believe.

Birch helps individuals to feel their roots, specifically their connection to family and ancestors. Birch is a tree that stands tall and firm and assists others in doing the same. It assists in overcoming negative generational patterns, especially in situations where one is at risk of being rejected if they choose a different way. It lends its spirit of endurance to help individuals face trials of adversity, so they may weather storms with the strength and conviction of a tree.

Birch teaches there is more to life than pain, and that with the right support and the right grounding, one can be held up and sustained by Divine grace.

Emotions Addressed: Unsupported, alienated, fear, weak-willed, overly flexible

Companion Oils: White Fir, Birch, Wintergreen, Grounding Blend

Black Pepper
The Oil of Unmasking

Black Pepper reveals the masks and façades used to hide aspects of the Self. Since childhood, most individuals have been taught that some feelings and behaviors are "good" while others are not. So instead of seeking to understand seemingly inappropriate feelings and behaviors, they usually judge, condemn and repress them. Individuals learn early on that to be loved and accepted they must hide undesirable aspects of themselves behind a mask or façade.

Black Pepper invites individuals to "get real" by digging deep within the less understood parts of the Self. Whether one's *true* motives and feelings are acknowledged or not, they continue to exist. The more these feelings are pushed down, buried and repressed, the more they seek to make themselves known. If they are not honestly dealt with and acknowledged, they will often be expressed through erratic, compulsive or addictive behaviors.

Black Pepper also re-ignites the soul fire, fueling motivation, high energy and hastening the healing process. It gives an individual strength to overcome the challenges and issues they carry inside and invites them to live in integrity with the Self.

Emotions Addressed: Emotional dishonesty, repressed emotions, feeling trapped, prideful, superficial, judgmental

Companion Oils: Vetiver, Frankincense, Cinnamon, Lavender

Cardamom
The Oil of Objectivity

Cardamom helps individuals to regain objectivity, mental sobriety and self-control. It assists individuals who frequently feel frustrated or angry with other people. Cardamom is especially helpful for times when one's anger goes to their head causing them to become "hot headed." In such situations, the individual becomes inebriated with anger, losing control and rational function. Cardamom helps to bring balance, mental clarity and objectivity during moments of extreme anger and frustration.

Cardamom is especially beneficial for individuals with a long history of anger or aggression, which often becomes directed outward. It is helpful for those who hyper-focus on their problems, especially their frustrations. Cardamom assists individuals to break down or "digest" these intense emotions of frustration and anger, by redirecting energy to the solar plexus, the center of responsibility. In this way Cardamom helps individuals let go of emotional distortions which cause them to objectify other people and see them as inconveniences.

Cardamom demands that individuals stop blaming others. It asks them to take personal ownership and responsibility for their feelings. As they do they will feel more at peace, calm and in control of themselves.

Emotions Addressed: Inebriated by anger, easily frustrated, objectifying others, blaming, unable to think clearly

Companion Oils: Thyme, Oregano, Digestive Blend, Calming Blend, Geranium

Cassia
The Oil of Self-Assurance

Cassia brings gladness and courage to the heart and soul. It is a wonderful remedy for the shy and timid. It helps those who hold back and try to hide. When a person avoids being the center of attention, Cassia can restore their confidence.

Similar to Cinnamon, Cassia dispels fear and replaces it with self-assurance. It challenges an individual to try, even when they are afraid of making mistakes. Cassia aids those who feel foolish by helping them see their own brilliance. It supports the soul in seeing its own value and potential. Cassia assists the individual in discovering their innate gifts and talents. It invites one to "let their light shine" and live from their authentic Self.

Emotions Addressed: Embarrassed, hiding, fear, humiliated, insecure, judged, shy, worthless

Companion Oils: Clove, Bergamot, Lavender, Melissa

Cedarwood

The Oil of Community

Cedarwood brings people together to experience the strength and value of community. Those in need of Cedarwood struggle to form bonds within social groups. This can often be due to an over-developed sense of individuality. Rather than allowing oneself to be supported by family, friends, or a community, they live by excessive self-reliance. On the other hand, the individual's difficulty forming social roots may also stem from feeling disconnected and separate from the human family. Cedarwood inspires the feeling of belonging and assists the heart in opening to receive the love and support of other people. It invites the strong willed individual to couple the strength of individuality with the supportive power of community.

Cedarwood supports individuals in seeing that they are not alone; life is a *shared* experience. Cedarwood also assists in opening the awareness of individuals to the support system that is already available to them, such as friends or family that have been overlooked. It invites individuals to both give and receive, so they may experience the strength of groups and the joy of relationships.

Emotions Addressed: Inability to form bonds or social roots, loneliness, feeling disconnected or separate from the human family, antisocial

Companion Oils: Marjoram, Birch, White Fir, Grounding Blend

Cilantro
The Oil of Releasing Control

Cilantro facilitates a detoxification of negative emotions and debris. It is helpful in lightening one's load through the release of issues buried in the body, heart and soul. Similar to Coriander oil, which is distilled from the seeds of the same plant, Cilantro assists individuals in shedding what is not in harmony with their True Self.

Those in need of Cilantro may attempt to obsessively control other people or manage their environment. Inwardly, these individuals may experience a great deal of worry and mental strain. The person may become constricted, clinging to or obsessing over material possessions. The individual may even hold onto the very patterns, emotions, issues and possessions which may impair or betray their True Self.

Cilantro facilitates emotional cleansing, and especially encourages the release of worry and control as it assists individuals in centering in their True Self. Cilantro liberates the soul from heavy burdens, enabling the individual to live light and free.

Emotions Addressed: Controlling, toxic, constricted, obsessive, clingy, emotionally trapped

Companion Oils: Coriander, Thyme, Cleansing Blend, Cypress, Cinnamon

Cinnamon

The Oil of Sexual Harmony

Cinnamon supports the reproductive system and helps heal sexual issues. It assists individuals in accepting their body and embracing their physical attractiveness. Cinnamon dispels fear of rejection and nurtures healthy sexuality. It rekindles sexual energies when there has been repression, trauma or abuse. It can also bring clarity to souls who struggle with their sexual identity.

Cinnamon also assists individuals in relationships where insecurities are shown by jealousy or control. It encourages the soul to let go of control and allow others to be free. Cinnamon can nurture strong relationships based on mutual love and respect.

Where there are other insecurities covered by pretense, façade and pride, Cinnamon invites individuals to be honest and vulnerable, thereby allowing true intimacy to emerge.

Emotions Addressed: Body rejection, fear, controlling, jealousy, sexual abuse, sexual repression or over-active sexuality

Companion Oils: Grapefruit, Metabolic Blend, Black Pepper, Focus Blend, Cilantro, Patchouli

Clary Sage
The Oil of Clarity & Vision

Clary Sage assists individuals in changing their perceptions. It gives courage to "see" the truth. One of the finest oils for the brow chakra, Clary Sage dispels darkness and illusion, helping a person to see their limiting belief systems. Clary Sage encourages individuals to remain open to new ideas and new perspectives. It can assist during a healing crisis when a drastic change of perspective is required. Clary Sage opens the soul to new possibilities and experiences.

Clary Sage assists in opening creative channels and clearing creative blocks. It eliminates distractions from the mind and assists individuals in finding a state of "emptiness" where creative forces may be realized. Opening them to the dream world, Clary Sage increases one's ability to visualize and imagine new possibilities.

Clary Sage teaches the spirit how to use its divinely given gifts and is especially helpful in clarifying spiritual vision. It assists in developing the gift of discernment. Clary Sage invites individuals to expand their vision and accept the reality of the spiritual world.

Emotions Addressed: Confusion, darkness, discouragement, disconnection from spiritual realms, hopeless, blocked creativity

Companion Oils: Lemongrass, Black Pepper, Melissa, Frankincense, Anti-Aging Blend

Clove

The Oil of Boundaries

Clove supports individuals in letting go of victim mentality. Victims feel overly influenced by other people and outside circumstances. They perceive themselves as powerless to change their life situations. Clove helps individuals to stand up for themselves, be proactive, and feel capable of making their own decisions, regardless of others' opinions or responses.

Clove assists individuals in letting go of patterns of self-betrayal and codependency by reconnecting them with their personal integrity. It builds up appropriate boundaries and defenses.

Clove gives the pushover the courage to say "no." It reignites the inner soul-fire and can assist anytime there has been damage to the Self, related to childhood pain, trauma or abuse. Clove is especially helpful for breaking free of patterns of abuse by restoring the victim's sense of Self and helping them regain the strength to stand up for their needs. Clove insists that individuals live true to themselves and the Divine by establishing clear boundaries.

Emotions Addressed: Victim, defeated, dominated, enslaved, fear of rejection, intimidated, controlled by others, co-dependent

Companion Oils: Ginger, Birch, Black Pepper, Protective Blend, Melaleuca

Coriander

The Oil of Loyalty

Coriander is the oil of loyalty, specifically loyalty to oneself. The person in need of Coriander oil may be trapped in a cycle of serving others while neglecting their own needs. They may also have a strong need to do what is right or correct. Often the mind's perspective of the "right" way is too limited and seen from only one perspective. Coriander reminds individuals that there is more than one way to do something, and that fitting in often requires betraying the True Self.

Coriander moves the individual from doing things for the acceptance of others to honoring and living from the True Self. There are as many ways of being as there are people in the world. Each soul must learn its own way of living and being. Coriander gives courage to step out of "the box" and risk being who one really is.

Coriander teaches that each individual is a gift to the world with something unique, which no one else has to offer. Only we can be and express our uniqueness. Loyalty to the Self means living in connection with what one's spirit urges and directs. Coriander shifts individuals from needing others' acceptance to honoring and living from the True Self.

Emotions Addressed: Controlled by others, self-betrayal, drudgery, conforming

Companion Oils: Frankincense, Cilantro, Lavender, Roman Chamomile, Detoxification Blend

Cypress
The Oil of Motion & Flow

This powerful oil creates energetic flow and emotional catharsis. Stagnant energies are brought into motion through the fluid energy of this oil. Cypress works in the heart and mind, creating flexibility.

Cypress teaches the soul how to let go of the past by moving with the flow of life. This oil is especially indicated for individuals who are mentally or emotionally stuck, stiff, rigid, tense, over-striving or have perfectionistic tendencies. This "hard-driving" stems from fear and the need to control. The individual tries to force things in life rather than allowing them to unfold naturally.

Cypress encourages individuals to cast aside their worries and let go of control so they can enjoy the thrill that comes from being alive. It reminds individuals that "damnation" is simply the discontinuation of growth and development. Cypress shows how to have perfect trust in the flow of life.

Emotions Addressed: Controlling, fear, perfectionism, rigidity, stuck, tense

Companion Oils: Peppermint, Cilantro, Vetiver, Massage Blend, Thyme

Eucalyptus

The Oil of Wellness

The strong medicinal aroma of Eucalyptus demonstrates its powerful effect upon the physical and emotional bodies. Eucalyptus oil supports the soul who is constantly facing illness. They may get well for times and seasons, only to return to a common cold, allergies or congestion in the sinuses and respiratory system.

Eucalyptus addresses a deep emotional or spiritual issue of the need to be sick. It reveals patterns of thinking that continually create poor health. Such beliefs may include thoughts like "I don't deserve to be well," "I am the sort of person that is always getting sick," or "The only way I can get a break is to get sick." Eucalyptus gives an individual courage to face these issues and beliefs. It encourages them to let go of their attachments to illness.

Eucalyptus encourages individuals to take full responsibility for their own health. It also bestows trust that one's needs and desires can be met, even if they allow themselves to be well. Eucalyptus teaches individuals how to claim their wholeness and heal.

Emotions Addressed: Attached to illness, clingy, defeated, despair, desire to escape life or responsibilities, imprisoned, powerless to heal, sickly

Companion Oils: Respiratory Blend, DNA Repairing Blend, Helichrysum

Fennel
The Oil of Responsibility

Fennel supports the individual who has a weakened sense of Self. The individual may feel defeated by life's responsibilities, having little to no desire to improve their situation. Fennel reignites a passion for life. It encourages the soul to take full ownership and responsibility for its choices. Fennel teaches that life is not too much or too big to handle.

Fennel encourages an individual to live in integrity with themselves, despite the judgments of others. When one has been paralyzed by fear and shame, this oil gets them moving again. Fennel re-establishes a strong connection to the body and the Self when there has been weakness or separation.

Fennel also supports an individual in listening to the subtle messages of the body. This is especially important in situations where there has been a loss of connection to the body's natural signals due to emotional eating, severe dieting, eating disorders or drug abuse. Through attunement with the body's actual needs, Fennel curbs cravings for experiences that dull the senses. This oil then supports the individual in hearing the body's signals of hunger, thirst, satiation, tiredness, or exhaustion. Fennel is also supportive in regaining one's appetite for nourishment, food and life itself.

Emotions Addressed: Lack of desire, unwilling to take responsibility for self or life, shame, weak sense of Self, numb to body signals

Companion Oils: Digestive Blend, Grapefruit, Ginger, Joyful Blend

Frankincense
The Oil of Truth

Frankincense reveals deceptions and false truths. It invites individuals to let go of lower vibrations, lies, deceptions and negativity. This oil helps create new perspectives based on light and truth. Frankincense recalls to memory spiritual understanding, gifts, wisdom and knowledge the soul brought into the world. It is a powerful cleanser of spiritual darkness. Frankincense assists in pulling the "scales of darkness" from the eyes, the barriers from the mind and the walls from the heart. Through connecting the soul with its inner light, this oil reveals the truth.

Frankincense supports in creating a healthy attachment with one's father. It assists in spiritual awakening and helps an individual feel the fatherly love of the Divine. When one has felt abandoned or forgotten, Frankincense reminds them that they are loved and protected. While this oil is incredibly powerful, it is also gentle, like a loving father who nurtures, guides and protects. Frankincense shields the body and soul from negative influences and assists the soul in its spiritual evolution. Enhancing practices of prayer and meditation, this oil opens spiritual channels that allow an individual to connect to God. Through the light and power of Frankincense, the individual can draw closer to divinity, healthy masculinity and the grandeur of the True Self.

Emotions Addressed: Abandonment, spiritually disconnected, distant from father, unprotected, spiritual darkness

Companion Oils: Myrrh, Roman Chamomile, Clary Sage, Melissa, Anti-Aging Blend, DNA Repairing Blend

Geranium
The Oil of Love & Trust

Geranium restores confidence in the innate goodness of others and in the world. It facilitates trust, especially when an individual has lost trust in others due to difficult life circumstances. It also assists in re-establishing a strong bond to one's mother and father. When there has been a loss of trust in relationships, geranium encourages emotional honesty, love and forgiveness. It fosters receptivity to human love and connection.

Geranium heals the broken heart. It encourages emotional honesty by facilitating the emergence of grief or pain that has been suppressed. Geranium softens anger and assists in healing emotional wounds. It assists in re-opening the heart so that love may flow freely. Indeed, Geranium could be called "the emotional healer."

Geranium is a gentle oil, perfect for babies and children. It nurtures the inner-child and supports in re-parenting this aspect of the Self. The individual who has a difficult time accessing their emotions can be supported by Geranium, as it leads away from the logical mind and into the warmth and nurture of the heart. At its root, Geranium heals the heart, instills unconditional love and fosters trust.

Emotions Addressed: Addresses almost all types of emotional issues, including: abandonment, loss, distrusting, unforgiving, unloving, disheartened, heavy hearted, grief, etc.

Companion Oils: Marjoram, Ylang Ylang, Rose, Calming Blend

Ginger
The Oil of Empowerment

Ginger oil holds no reservations. It has a purpose and it will fulfill it! Ginger powerfully persuades individuals to be fully present and participate in life. It teaches that to be successful in life one must be fully committed to it.

Ginger addresses deep patterns of victim mentality. A victim mentality is evidenced by feelings of powerlessness, believing everything is outside one's control, refusing to take responsibility for life, or blaming life circumstances on other people or outside influences. The victim feels stuck, as they decentralize or disown responsibility and blame others for their misfortunes.

Ginger empowers individuals in taking complete responsibility for their life circumstances. It infuses a warrior-like mentality based on personal integrity, centralized responsibility and individual choice. Here, the individual sees themselves as the creator of their own life. No longer waiting for outside circumstances to change, they choose their own destiny. The empowered individual assumes full responsibility and accountability for the consequences of their actions or inactions.

Emotions Addressed: Victim, powerless, unwilling to take responsibility for self or life, defeated, not present, stuck, blaming

Companion Oils: Clove, Fennel, Helichrysum, Protective Blend, Melaleuca

Grapefruit
The Oil of Honoring the Body

Grapefruit teaches true respect and appreciation for one's physical body. It supports individuals who struggle to honor their physical body and are caught in patterns of mistreatment. These forms of abuse may include severe dieting, judging one's body weight or type and abusing the body through negligent behavior or violence. These acts are often motivated by a hate and disgust buried within the psyche which gets directed toward the physical body. Though the individual may obsess over how they look, deep down they never feel they look good enough. There is a dissatisfaction that persists.

Grapefruit oil is often misused in overly strict dietary and weight-loss programs. The reason this oil helps curb emotional eating is because it encourages a positive relationship with one's physical body based on love, tolerance and acceptance. Grapefruit encourages integrity by respecting one's physical needs. This oil assists an individual in listening to their true physical needs and impulses. It also assists one in taking responsibility for what they feel. Grapefruit teaches that no amount of food can fill a hole in the heart - only love can do that. As the individual takes ownership of their feelings and gets the help they need in addressing them, they no longer have a need to hide their feelings behind food, body abuse, strict regimens, eating disorders or other forms of addiction.

Emotions Addressed: Hate for the body, addiction to food or dieting, eating disorders, anxiety over appearance

Companion Oils: Patchouli, Fennel, Metabolic Blend, Focus Blend

Helichrysum
The Oil for Pain

Helichrysum removes pain quickly and effortlessly. It aids "the walking wounded" – those with a history of difficult life circumstances, trauma, addiction, loss or abuse. These individuals need the powerful spiritual support that Helichrysum offers. It gives strength and endurance to the wounded soul who must keep on living, despite past difficulties. This oil restores confidence in life and in the Self, giving the individual strength to "make it." Helichrysum has a powerful relationship with the light of the sun. It imbues joy, fervor and hope for living. Helichrysum takes the wounded soul by the hand, guiding them through life's difficulties. If the wounded individual can persevere, this oil can take them into new heights of spiritual consciousness. Helichrysum offers hope that their wounds can be healed.

Following this spiritual healing and transformation, Helichrysum can teach an individual to have gratitude for their trials. It helps one to see that if they had not been wounded, they would not have sought healing that resulted in a spiritual rebirth. Just as the phoenix dies and is raised from its ashes, so might an individual be raised from their turmoil. Helichrysum lends its warrior spirit so that one may face their adversities with courage and determination. It brings hope to the most discouraged of souls and life to those in need of rebirth.

Emotions Addressed: Intense pain, anguish, turmoil, hopeless, despair, trauma, wounded

Companion Oils: Soothing Blend, Anti-Aging Blend, Ginger, Wintergreen

Jasmine
The Oil of Sexual Purity & Balance

Jasmine nurtures healthy sexuality and helps to balance sexual forces. It may also arouse dormant passions, assisting individuals to regain interest in the sexual experience. Jasmine cultivates positive experiences within intimate relationships by encouraging the purification of unhealthy sexual intentions and motivations. It asks individuals to honor and respect themselves and others.

Jasmine encourages the release of past sexual trauma. Through its gentle, purifying nature, Jasmine brings forward unresolved sexual experiences and facilitates the healing process. Traumatic experiences can distort one's relationship with sexuality. Jasmine can assist both kinds of common compensations: those who fear, repel or resist the sexual experience, as well as those who obsess over or are addicted to sexuality. It is balancing for individuals who use sex to fill a desperate need for love and approval, as well as individuals who resist sexual intimacy.

Jasmine supports the resolution of sexual trauma, encourages safety within intimate relationships, and invites only the purest intentions to the sexual experience.

Emotions Addressed: Unresolved sexual trauma, resistance to sexuality, sexual addiction

Companion Oils: Cinnamon, Ylang Ylang, Rose, Geranium

Juniper Berry
The Oil of Night

Juniper Berry assists those who fear the dark or unknown aspects of themselves. It helps individuals to understand that those things they fear are intended to be their teachers. Instead of hiding from what they do not understand, Juniper Berry encourages individuals to learn the lesson and face their fear. These fears often live within the unexplored areas of the Self. Juniper Berry acts as a catalyst by helping individuals access and address those fears and issues which have long been avoided.

Dreams contain nighttime communications. Even nightmares can reveal unresolved fears and issues. Juniper Berry offers courage and energetic protection in the nighttime. It encourages an honest assessment of the information being communicated from within.

As individuals reconcile with their fears and other hidden aspects of themselves they experience greater wholeness. Juniper helps restore the balance between light and dark, conscious and subconscious, day and night. It acts as a guide on the path toward wholeness. Juniper Berry teaches that there is truly nothing to fear when one acknowledges and accepts all aspects of the Self.

Emotions Addressed: Irrational fears, recurrent nightmares, restless sleep

Companion Oils: Black Pepper, Clary Sage, Vetiver

Lavender

The Oil of Communication

Lavender aids verbal expression. It calms the insecurities that are felt when one risks their true thoughts and feelings. Lavender addresses a deep fear of being seen and heard. Individuals in need of Lavender hide within, blocking all forms of true self-expression. While they may even be going through the motions of outward expression, they're actually holding back their innermost thoughts and feelings. The expression is not connected to the heart or soul.

Lavender supports individuals in releasing the tension and constriction that stems from fear of expressing one's Self. Due to past experiences, they may believe it is not safe to express themselves. The True Self is therefore trapped within and goes unexpressed. Strong feelings of being unlovable, unimportant, or unheard can accompany this condition. The individual's fear of rejection paralyzes their true voice and traps their feelings inside.

Lavender encourages emotional honesty and insists that one speak their innermost thoughts and desires. As individuals learn to communicate their deepest thoughts and feelings, they are liberated from their self-inflicted prison. It is through open and honest communication that an individual experiences unconditional love and acceptance. Through Lavender's courageous spirit, one is free to share their True Self with others.

Emotions Addressed: Blocked communication, fear of rejection, feeling unseen or unheard, constricted, tension, emotional dishonesty, hiding, fear of self-disclosure

Companion Oils: Lime, Cassia, Monthly Blend

Lemon
The Oil of Focus

The delightful citrusy aroma of Lemon oil nourishes the mind and aids concentration. While Lemon supports the emotional body, its major effects are experienced in the mental field. The crisp scent of Lemon oil improves one's ability to focus. Lemon is a wonderful aid for children struggling with school. It teaches individuals to be mentally present by focusing on one thing at a time. Lemon dispels confusion and bestows clarity. It counterbalances mental fatigue due to too much studying or reading. Lemon restores energy, mental flexibility and the drive to complete a project.

Lemon is especially helpful in cases of learning disorders. Whether an individual has a difficult time concentrating or feels incapable of learning, Lemon clears self-judgments about learning such as "I'm dumb" or "I am not a good student." Lemon calms fears and insecurities while restoring confidence in the Self.

Emotionally, Lemon inspires a natural playfulness and buoyancy in the heart. It assists in releasing feelings of depression by restoring feelings of joy and happiness. Lemon inspires joyful involvement in the present moment by infusing the soul with energy, confidence and alertness.

Emotions Addressed: Confusion, inability to focus, mental fatigue, lack of joy and energy, learning disorders, guilt

Companion Oils: Rosemary, Digestive Blend, Invigorating Blend, Joyful Blend

Lemongrass
The Oil of Cleansing

Lemongrass is a powerful cleanser of energy. It dispels feelings of despondency, despair and lethargy. Lemongrass assists individuals in entering a healing mode or cleansing state. In this state, one easily lets go of old, limiting beliefs, toxic energies and negativity. Lemongrass teaches individuals to move forward without hesitation. It asks them to commit to a healing path where change is a regular occurrence.

Lemongrass can also be a powerful tool in cleansing the energy within a house, room or office space. It encourages individuals with pack-rat tendencies to courageously let go of everything they no longer need.

Lemongrass also clears negative energy from the brow chakra or spiritual eyes. As individuals lets go of past issues and stagnant energy, they have an increased ability to see situations with greater clarity. It supports individuals' energy in flowing freely and smoothly. Lemongrass has a powerful mission to assist in cleansing physically, emotionally and spiritually.

Emotions Addressed: Toxic or negative energy, despair, holding on to the past, hoarding, darkness, spiritual blindness

Companion Oils: Cleansing Blend, Melaleuca, Thyme, Clary Sage, Detoxification Blend, DNA Repairing Blend

Lime
The Oil of Zest for Life

Lime imbues the soul with a zest for life. When an individual has been weighed down by discouragement or grief, Lime elevates them above the mire. It instills courage and cheer in the heart and reminds them to be grateful for the gift of life.

Lime cleanses the heart, especially when there has been an accumulation of emotional toxins due to avoidance or repression. This oil revitalizes the heart space, giving room for light and joy. It clears discouragement, depression and suicidal thoughts and feelings. Lime shines light on the inner motives hidden in the heart and encourages emotional honesty.

Lime can also assist the individual who has overly developed their intellectual capacities but has neglected to develop themselves emotionally. This oil encourages balance between the heart and mind. It clears congestion from the heart region, assisting one in feeling safe and at home in their heart. Lime dispels apathy and resignation and instills hope, joy, courage and the determination to face all of life's challenges.

Emotions Addressed: Apathy, resignation, grief, suicidal thoughts and feelings, discouragement

Companion Oils: Tangerine, Joyful Blend, Melissa, Invigorating Blend

Marjoram

The Oil of Connection

Marjoram aids those who are unable to trust others or form meaningful relationships. This inability to trust often stems from harsh life experiences. The individual develops a fear of close connection in human relationships. They may tend towards reclusive behaviors, protecting themselves even further by abstaining from social interactions. They may also protect themselves by unconsciously sabotaging long-term relationships. Marjoram shows the barriers they have formed to protect themselves from others. It reveals patterns of aloofness, distancing one's self from other people, or being "cold." Those in need of Marjoram oil most likely use these protective coping strategies unintentionally. Deep down they desire the intimate connection they subconsciously sabotage.

Marjoram teaches that trust is the basis for all human relationships. It assists an individual in increasing their warmth and trust in social situations. Marjoram softens the heart and heals past wounds. It kindles the fires of trust in relationships so that one may fully blossom. When an individual feels safe and loved, they express their authenticity more freely. Marjoram restores trust and openness so that true bonds of love may be formed in friendships and relationships.

Emotions Addressed: Distrust, aloof, protected, distant, emotional isolation, reclusive, emotionally "cold," fear of rejection

Companion Oils: Cedarwood, Monthly Blend, Calming Blend, Geranium, Women's Blend

Melaleuca
The Oil of Energetic Boundaries

Disinfectant by nature, Melaleuca, also known as tea tree oil, clears negative energetic baggage. It specifically releases codependent and parasitic relationships. These toxic relationships may be with people, microorganisms in the physical body, or spiritual beings. The individual may feel drained of life force and energy, but they may not be consciously aware of the source of this energy leakage. Melaleuca helps break the negative ties in these kinds of relationships so that new, healthy connections may be formed that honor one's personal space and boundaries. This energetic "vampirism" between organisms violates the laws of nature. Melaleuca encourages an individual to connect to people and beings in ways that honor and respect others' agency. It helps the individual to recognize the parts of themselves that invited and allowed these kinds of relationships to exist in the first place.

Through these empowering processes, Melaleuca encourages an individual to relinquish all forms of self-betrayal, including: allowing others to take advantage of one's time, energy or talents; letting others feed on one's energy; not standing up for oneself; or feeling responsible for the problems of others. Melaleuca assists individuals in purification practices and in releasing toxic debris.

Emotions Addressed: Parasitic and codependent relationships, poor boundaries, weak willed, toxicity

Companion Oils: Thyme, Oregano, Lemongrass, Cleansing Blend

Melissa
The Oil of Light

Melissa oil awakens the soul to truth and light. It reminds individuals of who they truly are and why they came to this earth. Melissa invites one to release everything and anything that holds them back from reaching their fullest potential.

Melissa assists an individual in receiving spiritual guidance by reconnecting them with their inner voice. It uplifts the soul by literally preparing one to "up-level." When an individual feels too weighed down by the burdens of life, Melissa encourages them to keep going. It gives strength and vitality to the innermost recesses of the heart and soul. This oil invites one to participate in higher realms of living and dreaming. As an individual stays connected to spiritual sources, they feel a lightness in their being and a brightness in their core. Melissa reminds one that every individual has a spark of divinity within them and that with love and attention, that spark will grow. This oil fuels that spark of energy, igniting an individual's True Self. Melissa assists them in shedding everything that is not in harmony with their inner light.

Melissa's enthusiasm is contagious. Through the intense light and vibration Melissa has to offer, an individual may feel they cannot help but let go of depression and other low vibrations that are holding them down. It teaches one the joy of living.

Emotions Addressed: Depression, darkened, dreary, suicidal, overwhelmed

Companion Oils: Lime, Tangerine, Joyful Blend, Anti-Aging Blend, Invigorating Blend

Myrrh
The Oil of Mother Earth

Myrrh oil nurtures the soul's relationship with it's maternal mother and with the earth. This oil supports individuals who have had disturbances with the mother-child bond. Whether it is a division between the child and the biological mother or whether it be mother earth herself, Myrrh can help bridge the gap and heal the disturbance. This division or lack of attachment may be related to adoption, birth trauma, malnourishment, experiences of abandonment, or other childhood issues. Myrrh helps the soul to feel the love and nurturing presence of "Mother." Similar to the nutrient-rich colostrum found in a mother's milk, Myrrh oil inoculates individuals from the adverse and harmful effects of the world. Like the warmth of a mother's love for her child, Myrrh assists individuals in feeling safe and secure.

When the mother-child bond has been disrupted, the soul may lose its childlike ability to trust. Feelings of trust are replaced with feelings of fear and a belief that the world is unsafe. Myrrh assists individuals in letting go of fear. Through reestablishing a healthy connection to the earth and to one's own mother, Myrrh rekindles trust within the soul. As the individual learns to once again live in trust, confidence in the goodness of life returns and the soul feels more safe and at home on the earth.

Emotions Addressed: Disrupted maternal connection, distrust of others, feeling unsafe in the world, malnourished

Companion Oils: Women's Blend, Monthly Blend, Frankincense, Grounding Blend

Oregano

The Oil of Humility & Non-Attachment

Oregano cuts through the fluff of life and teaches individuals to do the same. It removes blocks, clears negativity and cuts away negative attachments. Oregano is a powerful oil and may even be described as forceful or intense.

Oregano addresses a person's need to be "right." The individual in need of Oregano may attempt to convert other people to their own fixed opinions. Their strong will can make them unteachable and unwilling to budge. They hold rigidly to their opinions and belief systems. However, Oregano is resolute and has the power to break through a strong will.

On the deepest level, Oregano dispels materialism and attachment that hinders an individual's growth and progress. While using Oregano, a person may feel encouraged to end a toxic relationship, quit an oppressive job, or end a lifelong addiction. These toxic attachments limit one's capacity to feel a healthy connection to the Divine. Oregano encourages true spirituality by inviting the soul to live in non-attachment. It teaches that devotion to one's Higher Power includes letting go of rigidity, willfulness, negative attachments and materialism.

Emotions Addressed: Overly attached, pride, opinionated, negative, excessively willful, materialistic

Companion Oils: Sandalwood, Thyme, Melaleuca, Lemongrass, Detoxification Blend

Patchouli
The Oil of Physicality

Patchouli supports individuals in becoming fully present in their physical body. It balances those who feel devitalized and who seek to escape the body through spiritual pursuits or other forms of distraction. Patchouli tempers the obsessive personality by bringing them "down" to reality and teaching them moderation. It is grounding and stabilizing.

Patchouli compliments yoga practice, tai chi, or other exercises that aim to connect the spirit with the body. While using Patchouli, individuals feel more grounded and fluid. This oil calms fears and nervous tension, stilling the heart and mind in preparing the spirit and body for deeper union. It also helps individuals to stay in touch with the earth.

Patchouli helps individuals to appreciate the magnificence of the physical body and all of its natural processes and functions. It assists in releasing emotional judgments and issues related to the body, such as believing the body is unholy or dirty. This oil helps with body image distortions and general body dislike. Patchouli brings confidence in the body, as well as grace, poise and physical strength. It reminds individuals of their childhood experiences when they used their bodies for play and fun. On the deepest level, Patchouli assists an individual to feel at peace while being present in their physical body.

Emotions Addressed: Body shame, disconnect from the body, judgment of the body, tension in body

Companion Oils: Focus Blend, Grapefruit, Cinnamon, Metabolic Blend, Grounding Blend

Peppermint
The Oil of a Buoyant Heart

Peppermint brings joy and buoyancy to the heart and soul. It invigorates body, mind and spirit and reminds individuals that life can be happy and there is nothing to fear. It lifts an individual out of their emotional trials for a short reprieve. When an individual uses Peppermint, they feel as though they're gliding through life. It assists in staying on the surface of emotional issues like a water skier on a lake.

The power of Peppermint can be felt most in times of discouragement or depression. When the individual is disheartened, they may use Peppermint to re-discover the joy of being alive.

However, a person may also abuse the properties of Peppermint oil. If it is used as a permanent escape to avoid dealing with emotional pain, it can hinder growth and progress. Peppermint should not be used in this way. It aids individuals who need a short "breather." At times, a reprieve is necessary before re-entering emotional waters, but we are not meant to wade in the shallow end forever. When it is accepted and embraced, emotional pain serves as a teacher. Peppermint can assist an individual in regaining the strength needed to face their emotional reality.

Emotions Addressed: Unbearable pain, intense depression, heaviness, pessimistic, muddled

Companion Oils: Joyful Blend, Tangerine, Lime, Rose, Cypress

Roman Chamomile
The Oil of Spiritual Purpose

Roman Chamomile supports an individual in discovering and living their true life purpose. Regardless of what they do for a living, Chamomile helps them find purpose and meaning in their lives. As individuals live from the center of their beings, they find a power and a purpose that is indescribable. They feel more at peace and more calm. Chamomile softens the personality, easing the overactive ego-mind. It restores one's confidence to do what they came here to do. Like a guardian angel, Chamomile leads the soul to where it needs to be and what it needs to be doing.

Roman Chamomile assists a person in shedding the meaningless activities that consume their lives so that they can focus on a more fulfilling work, even the work of their own souls. Chamomile assists in feeling connected to and supported by divine helpers and guides. It calms insecurities about following one's spiritual path. People fear and believe that if they do what they love, they will end up destitute. Roman Chamomile says, "Do what you love and everything will be a success."

Emotions Addressed: Purposeless, discouraged, drudgery, frustration, unsettled

Companion Oils: Frankincense, Melissa, Anti-Aging Blend

Rose

The Oil of Divine Love

Rose oil holds a higher frequency than any other oil on the planet. It is a powerful healer of the heart. It supports an individual in reaching heavenward and contacting Divine love. Rose teaches the essential need for Divine grace and intervention in the healing process. As an individual opens to receive Divine benevolence in all its manifestations, the heart is softened. If one can simply let go and choose to receive Divine love, they are wrapped in warmth, charity and compassion.

Rose invites individuals to experience the unwavering, unchanging, unconditional love of the Divine. This love heals all hearts and dresses all wounds. It restores an individual to authenticity, wholeness and purity. As one feels unconditional love and acceptance, the heart is softened. As the heart is fully opened, a fountain of love flows freely through the soul. In this state, one feels charity and compassion. Charity is experienced on behalf of oneself and others. Rose embodies Divine love and teaches individuals how to contact this love through prayer, meditation and opening the heart to receive.

Emotions Addressed: Bereft of divine love, constricted feelings, closed or broken heart, lack of brotherly love

Companion Oils: Geranium, Ylang Ylang, Calming Blend, Thyme, Calming Blend, Monthly Blend

Rosemary
The Oil of Knowledge & Transition

Rosemary assists in the development of true knowledge and true intellect. It teaches that one can be instructed from a far greater space of understanding than the human mind. It challenges individuals to look deeper than they normally would and ask more soul-searching questions so that they may receive more inspired answers.

Rosemary assists individuals who struggle with learning disabilities. It brings expansion to the mind, supporting individuals in receiving new information and new experiences.

Rosemary aids in times of transition and change. When a person is having a difficult time adjusting to a new house, school, or relationship, Rosemary can assist. Rosemary teaches that we do not understand all things because we have a mortal perspective. It invites individuals to trust in a higher, more intelligent power than themselves. It supports them in feeling confident and assured during times of great change in understanding or perspective. Rosemary roots them in the true knowledge that surpasses all understanding.

Emotions Addressed: Confusion, difficulty adjusting or transitioning, ignorance, difficulties with learning

Companion Oils: Lemon, Digestive Blend, Detoxification Blend

Sandalwood
The Oil of Sacred Devotion

Sandalwood assists with all kinds of prayer, meditation and spiritual worship. It teaches reverence and respect for Deity. This oil has been used since ancient times for its powerful ability to calm the mind, still the heart and prepare the spirit to commune with God.

Sandalwood teaches of spiritual devotion and spiritual sacrifice. It invites individuals to place all material attachments on the altar of sacrifice so that they may truly progress spiritually. This oil asks individuals to assess where their hearts are and challenges them to reorder their priorities to be in alignment with the Divine will.

Sandalwood assists in quieting the mind so that individuals may hear the subtle voice of the Spirit. It raises them into higher levels of consciousness. Sandalwood assists one in reaching beyond their current confines and belief systems. For those who are ready to leave behind attachment to fame, wealth and the need for acceptance, Sandalwood teaches true humility, devotion and love for the Divine.

Emotions Addressed: Disconnected from God or spiritual Self, emptiness, over-thinking, materialism

Companion Oils: Oregano, Frankincense, Myrrh, Anti-Aging Blend

Tangerine
The Oil of Cheer & Creativity

Tangerine's strong qualities of cheer and joyfulness can lift the darkest of moods. It can assist those who feel cut off from the lightness of heart often manifested by children. Those who feel overburdened by responsibility would benefit from Tangerine's uplifting vibration. It encourages a person to be creative and spontaneous.

Creativity can be stifled by an excessive sense of duty or creating rigid standards for oneself. While work, duty and responsibility all have their place, feeling overworked, overly-responsible and overburdened leads to a loss of creative energy. Tangerine invites individuals to make room for their creative side. It asks that we reinsert fun, joy and spontaneity into our lives.

Tangerine supports an individual in accessing the abundant pool of creative energy held within the spirit. It then assists that energy in flowing through the heart and into physical manifestation. Tangerine teaches the individual to enjoy life by being more abundantly creative and to re-experience the joy and cheerfulness they knew in childhood.

Emotions Addressed: Overburdened by responsibilities, dutifulness which stifles creativity, downtrodden, heavy heart, lack of fun or joy in life

Companion Oils: Wild Orange, Ylang Ylang, Roman Chamomile, Lime, Invigorating Blend

Thyme
The Oil of Releasing & Forgiving

Thyme is one of the most powerful cleansers of the emotional body and assists in addressing trapped feelings which have been buried for a long time. It reaches deep within the body and soul, searching for unresolved negativity. Thyme brings to the surface old, stagnant feelings. It is particularly helpful in treating the toxic emotions of hate, rage, anger and resentment, which cause the heart to close.

Thyme empties the soul of all negativity, leaving the heart wide open. In this state of openness, an individual begins to feel tolerance and patience for others. As the heart opens more and more, it is able to receive love and offer forgiveness. Thyme teaches, "It's time to move forward and let go." As individuals forgive, they free themselves from emotional bondage. Thyme transforms hate and anger into love and forgiveness.

Emotions Addressed: Unforgiving heart, anger, rage, hate, bitterness, resentment, emotional bondage

Companion Oils: Cypress, Lemongrass, Detoxification Blend, Cleansing Blend

Vetiver
The Oil of Centering & Descent

Vetiver oil assists in becoming more rooted in life. Life can scatter one's energy and cause one to feel split between different priorities, people and activities. Vetiver brings the individual back down to earth. It assists them in grounding to the physical world. Vetiver also assists individuals in deeply connecting with what they think and feel. In this way, Vetiver is incredibly supportive in all kinds of self-awareness work. It helps uncover the root of an emotional issue.

Vetiver challenges individuals' need to escape their pain. It centers them in Self and guides them downward to the root of their emotional issues. It helps them find relief, but not through avoidance. Relief comes after they have traveled within and met the core of their emotional issue. Vetiver will not let them quit. It grounds them in the present moment and carries them through an emotional catharsis. The descent into the Self assists individuals in discovering deeper facets of their being. Vetiver opens the doors to light and recovery through this downward journey.

Emotions Addressed: Apathetic, despondent, disconnected, scattered, split, stressed, ungrounded, need to escape, crisis

Companion Oils: Black Pepper, Grounding Blend, Cypress, Focus Blend

White Fir

The Oil of Generational Healing

White Fir addresses generational issues. Patterns and traditions are passed down from family member to family member. Some of these patterns are positive, while others are negative and destructive. Examples of negative patterns may include: addiction, abuse, alcoholism, anger, codependency, eating disorders, pride, the need to be right, etc.

White Fir assists the individual in unearthing these negative patterns from the hidden recesses of the body and soul. As they are brought to the light of consciousness, they can be dealt with and put to rest. The individual can choose not to participate in destructive family patterns and thereby break the tradition. White Fir aids this process and increases an individual's chances of success. In breaking these patterns, it offers a refuge of spiritual protection and helps individuals stay true to the path of healing, even if their family members oppose them in leaving behind their traditions.

Emotions Addressed: Feelings that are generational or hereditary, burdened by the issues of others

Companion Oils: DNA Repairing Blend, Grounding Blend, Birch, Cedarwood

Wild Orange
The Oil of Abundance

Wild Orange addresses a wide variety of emotional issues. It inspires abundance, fosters creativity, supports a positive mood, restores physical energy and aids in transitions. Wild Orange also reconnects individuals with their inner child and brings spontaneity, fun, joy and play into one's life.

At its core, Wild Orange teaches the true meaning of abundance. It encourages individuals to let go of scarcity mindsets with all of their manifestations, including: fear, nervousness, inflexibility, workaholism, lack of humor and the belief that there is not enough. Wild Orange reminds the soul of the limitless supply found in nature. Fruit trees, like orange, give freely to all in need. Wild Orange teaches individuals to give without thought of compensation. In nature, there is always enough to go around. Wild Orange encourages individuals to let go of their need to hoard, which is the epitome of scarcity.

Wild Orange also assists an individual's natural creative sense. It inspires limitless solutions for problems and issues. One never needs to fear. Wild Orange invites the individual to completely let go as a child does and to live from their authentic Self. In our authenticity, we are abundance. Sharing, playing, relaxing and enjoying the bounties of life - these are the gifts bestowed by Wild Orange essential oil.

Emotions Addressed: Scarcity, over-serious, rigid, dull, workaholism, low energy, discouraged, hoarding, envy

Companion Oils: Tangerine, Ylang Ylang, Lemon, Peppermint

Wintergreen

The Oil of Surrender

Wintergreen is the oil of surrender. It can assist the strong-willed individual in letting go of the need to know and the need to be right. It takes great internal strength to surrender to one's Higher Power. Wintergreen imbues the soul with this strength and teaches it how to let go and be free of the negativity and pain it holds on to. The need to believe that life is painful and one must shoulder it on their own will make it so. Wintergreen invites individuals to surrender these strong opinions.

Yet, Wintergreen reminds individuals that they do not have to do life on their own. There is a constant invitation to surrender one's burdens to a Higher Power. All that is required is to release and let go. Wintergreen teaches that one can turn their hardships over to that Power greater than themselves so they do not have to carry the burden of life all alone.

Emotions Addressed: Need to control, feeling weak, willful, need to be right, holding on, excessive self-reliance

Companion Oils: Sandalwood, Oregano, Birch, Eucalyptus, Frankincense

Ylang Ylang
The Oil of the Inner Child

Ylang Ylang is a powerful remedy for the heart. Modern day society honors and reveres the mind over the heart. Yet the heart, with its intuitive ways of receiving information is an essential part of the soul. Ylang Ylang reconnects an individual with the child self and the pure, simple ways of the heart. It encourages play and restores a childlike nature and innocence. It assists in accessing intuition or "heart knowing."

Ylang Ylang is also a powerful remedy for releasing emotional trauma from the past. It is a fantastic support in age regression work and other methods of emotional healing. Ylang Ylang also assists individuals in releasing bottled up emotions such as anger and sadness. Feelings that have been buried inside are easily brought to the light through Ylang Ylang's assistance. This oil allows emotional healing to flow naturally, nurturing the heart through the process. It reminds the individual that joy can be felt and experienced more fully by allowing the heart its full range of emotions.

Emotions Addressed: Joylessness, overstressed, grief, sadness, loss of a loved one, disconnected from inner-child

Companion Oils: Calming Blend, Tangerine, Wild Orange, Rose, Geranium

OIL BLENDS

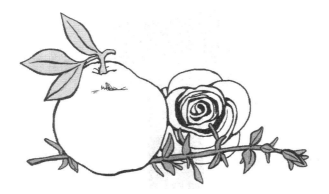

Introducing Oil Blends

How to Find Your Favorite Blend

As requested, we have not used any trademark names in the Oil Blends. However, most blends are listed by their sub-title name and can be easily found by looking at your bottle. For example, if the blend you are looking for is Breathe, then the subtitle is Respiratory Blend in this book.

About Oil Blends

Oil blends are created by combining several single oils to form an entirely new product. Blends are formulated to address a specific physical or emotional theme or issue. Oil blends are different from single oils but not necessarily superior. Still, blends may be more equipped than single oils in some ways. When oil blends are formulated well, they create synergies, or increased effectiveness, in supporting those specific issues they were created to address.

Anti-Aging Blend
The Oil of Spiritual Insight

Essential oils have been used since antiquity to assist meditation practices, prayer and spiritual worship. Anti-Aging Blend combines the power of high vibrational oils alongside grounding oils to assist the connection between spirit and body, heaven and earth. This blend encourages positive states of being and supports the development of faith, hope, gratitude, kindness, love, patience and trust in the Divine.

Anti-Aging Blend is a wonderful aid for meditation as it quiets the mind, fosters inner stillness and encourages spiritual growth. While this oil is gentle, it is also very powerful. It assists the release of negativity, darkness and limiting perceptions. Anti-Aging Blend can mitigate spiritual blindness and other spiritual issues by offering profound light to individuals.

Anti-Aging Blend offers grace and comfort when one feels discouraged or distressed. This oil can assist individuals in transcending the darkness, pain and stresses of life. At its core, Anti-Aging Blend offers support in raising levels of human consciousness and preparing individuals for new heights of spiritual transformation.

Ingredients: Frankincense, Sandalwood, Lavender, Myrrh and other essential oils

Emotions Addressed: Dark night of the soul, spiritual blindness, burdened, discouraged

Companion Oils: Frankincense, Helichrysum, Rose, Sandalwood, DNA Repairing Blend, Wintergreen

Calming Blend
The Oil of Forgiveness

Calming Blend has a powerful effect on the heart. It may calm feelings of hostility, fear, anger, jealousy, rage and resentment. Calming Blend can support individuals who struggle to forgive others for their hurtful blunders and behaviors. Combined, the oils of this blend soften the hardened heart and assist individuals in overcoming their criticisms and judgments of other people. When an individual expects too much from others, Calming Blend can relax their perfectionistic expectations. It assists individuals in viewing others with tenderness and compassion. It teaches that Divine grace is for all and that no one is perfect. The need to blame others stems from unhappiness and pain in one's own life. Calming Blend encourages individuals to look at themselves first when they feel like blaming someone else.

Calming Blend brings a person more in touch with the qualities of love, openness and receptivity. This blend helps heal the emotional wounds in the heart so that love may flow freely. Calming Blend fosters tenderness and love in every relationship. It assists the heart in remaining whole by practicing principles of forgiveness.

Ingredients: Lavender, Marjoram, Roman Chamomile, Ylang Ylang and other essential oils

Emotions Addressed: Resentment, unwillingness to forgive, bitterness, anger, sadness, criticism, perfectionism

Companion Oils: Geranium, Marjoram, Rose, Monthly Blend, Women's Blend, Ylang Ylang

Cleansing Blend
The Oil of Purification

Cleansing Blend assists individuals in releasing toxic emotions and entering a cleansing state. It revitalizes the energy system, washing away negative influences. This blend supports individuals who feel trapped by negativity or toxicity. Cleansing Blend provides freedom from past habits and patterns. It is especially helpful in combating toxic feelings of hate, rage and enmeshment and in severing other negative attachments.

Like Lemongrass, Cleansing Blend makes a wonderful space cleanser. It can clear negative energy from the household and the environment, as well as cleanse the air of odor and harmful microorganisms. Diffused in the air, this oil can facilitate emotional breakthroughs. In order to heal, we must receive. But in order to receive, we must first release what is blocking the new, clean energy from entering in. Cleansing Blend supports individuals in constantly releasing the old so they may be open to the new.

Ingredients: Lemon, Lime, Pine, Citronella and other essential oils

Emotions Addressed: Trapped, stuck, toxic emotions, negative attachments

Companion Oils: Lemongrass, Thyme, Cilantro, Detoxification Blend, DNA Repairing Blend

Detoxification Blend
The Oil of Vitality & Transition

Detoxification Blend is designed to cleanse the organs and systems of the body. Emotionally, this blend assists during times of transition and change. It can assist an individual in "detoxing" old habits and limiting beliefs. When an individual has felt trapped by self-sabotaging behaviors or addictions, Detoxification Blend paves the way for new life experiences. It aids in letting go of behaviors that are destructive to one's health and happiness. It is especially helpful during major life changes which require adjustments in habit and lifestyle, such as altering diet, quitting smoking, or leaving a toxic relationship.

Detoxification Blend reawakens vital life energy. It also assists an individual in discovering new energy and vitality by encouraging the release of physical and emotional toxins. This blend aids in shedding apathy as well as any destructive habit, helping a person find new enthusiasm for life. As individuals let go of limiting beliefs, behaviors and lifestyles, they have greater room to receive. As a result, they are able to see life from a fresh perspective and embrace new experiences.

Ingredients: Tangerine, Rosemary, Geranium and other essential oils

Emotions Addressed: Difficulty with transitions, addiction, toxic habits, limiting beliefs, apathy

Companion Oils: Lemongrass, Rosemary, Melaleuca, Cleansing Blend, DNA Repairing Blend, Cilantro

Digestive Blend
The Oil of Digestion

The Digestive Blend was formulated to support the body's digestive system. It also has a powerful emotional quality for supporting individuals who lack interest in life and the physical world. The individual may have a tendency to "bite off more than they can chew" by trying to do too much at once. This overload of information and stimulation may lead to an emotional form of "indigestion," where the individual cannot break down life experiences into palatable forms. The soul literally becomes overfed and undernourished, as it cannot translate its experiences into a usable form. When the individual is fully overwhelmed and over stimulated, they may lose their appetite for food, life and the physical world in general. They may become apathetic about their situation and begin neglecting their body's basic needs.

Digestive Blend combines the powerful oils of Ginger, Peppermint and other spices to support the body and the spirit in assimilating new information and events. It increases an individual's ability to receive new information, new relationships and new experiences and be open to new possibilities. This blend powerfully aids individuals in digesting life's many experiences.

Ingredients: Ginger, Peppermint, Tarragon, Fennel, Caraway and other essential oils

Emotions Addressed: Loss of appetite for food or life, inability to assimilate new information or experiences, over stimulated

Companion Oils: Rosemary, Fennel, Ginger, Lemon

DNA Repairing Blend
The Oil of Transformation

DNA Repairing Blend works emotionally as well as physically with the cycles of life and death and personal transformation. By putting off the old we become free to experience the new—this is transformation. DNA Repairing Blend supports the body's sick or damaged cells to either transition to death, or to transform, repair and renew. Through the help and support of this blend individuals can assist their bodies, cells, energy and emotions in returning to a balanced, healthy and authentic state.

DNA Repairing Blend is particularly supportive in releasing all types of negative family patterns which are recorded in the body itself (in the DNA). It is especially suited for those who struggle with debilitating circumstances, as it helps to relieve feelings of doubt, disbelief, despair, and burden. It teaches individuals to reclaim their life energy and to believe that change is possible. DNA Repairing Blend supports the process of regaining health and vitality by encouraging the release of the old, the birth of the new, and the cycles of life, death, and rebirth.

Ingredients: Frankincense, Wild Orange, Lemongrass, Thyme, Summer Savory and other essential oils

Emotions Addressed: Debilitated, discouraged, toxic, stuck, burdened by family patterns

Companion Oils: Eucalyptus, White Fir, Frankincense, Basil, Detoxification Blend

Focus Blend

The Oil of Presence

In contrast to Lemon oil, *The Oil of Focus*, Focus Blend calms the mind, facilitating inner peace. Whereas Lemon activates the mind, Focus Blend quiets and grounds mental forces. It is especially beneficial to those with a short attention span. It encourages individuals to remain present with the task at hand and to complete a project, goal or activity before moving onto the next. Focus Blend is therefore supportive to individuals who become lost in thought—those who rapidly jump from one activity or idea to the next—as well as those who lose themselves in daydreams or fantasy.

Focus Blend gently guides the soul into full awareness of its physical body and physical surroundings. It invites individuals to accept the reality of their life situation, so they may deal with it appropriately. This blend especially encourages individuals to live in the *here and now*, and therefore promotes a meditative state. Focus Blend's stability and grounding energy supports a healthy connection between the body and the mind. With the support of Focus Blend, individuals are empowered to live fully connected in the present moment.

Ingredients: Amyris, Patchouli, Frankincense, Lime, Ylang Ylang and other essential oils

Emotions Addressed: Distraction, lack of physical presence or awareness, daydreaming, procrastination, scattered

Companion Oils: Patchouli, Sandalwood, Vetiver, Grounding Blend

Grounding Blend
The Oil of Grounding

The Grounding Blend is primarily a combination of tree oils and roots. Trees live in the present moment. They are not in a hurry. They are stable. Grounding Blend's soft energy is excellent for calming hyperactive children who have difficulty settling down. It is also a wonderful remedy for adults who need to reconnect with their roots. Grounding Blend strengthens a connection with the lower body and with the earth. These connections are especially important when the upper faculties have been overused due to excessive thinking, speaking, or spiritual activity.

Grounding Blend is especially suited for personalities who seek to escape from life through disconnection or disassociation. These individuals may avoid long-term commitments in work or relationships, preferring instead to "drift" with the wind. This blend reminds individuals that to realize their true dreams and desires, they must stay focused on a goal until it is actualized in the physical world. Grounding Blend teaches true perseverance by assisting the individual in staying present with a specific plan or idea until it is embodied. Providing inner strength and fortitude, Grounding Blend teaches individuals to ground their energy and to manifest their vision with the patience of a tree.

Ingredients: Spruce, Ho Wood, Frankincense and other essential oils

Emotions Addressed: Ungrounded, unwilling to take responsibility for self or life, disconnected, unstable, scattered

Companion Oils: Focus Blend, Vetiver, Patchouli, Myrrh, Birch

Invigorating Blend
The Oil of Creativity

Invigorating Blend acts as a powerful "fire starter." It returns motivation and drive when it is lacking. This is a wonderful combination of oils for addressing lethargy, discouragement, despondency, or low will to live. When the soul has lost its connection to the magic in life, this blend helps restore the spark.

The Invigorating Blend also inspires creativity. Every human soul has a need to create. These oils inspire creative expression by reconnecting individuals with their inner child and their natural creative sense. They assist individuals in living abundantly and spontaneously by encouraging play and excitement. Invigorating Blend can motivate individuals to use their true creative power by letting go of old limitations and insecurities. It takes courage to put oneself out there artistically. Citruses in particular bring color and imagination to one's life. Placed over the solar plexus, this combination of oils restores confidence in one's Self and in one's creations. Invigorating Blend rekindles the fire of the personality and fills the heart with creativity and joy.

Ingredients: Wild Orange, Lemon, Grapefruit, Mandarin, Bergamot, Tangerine and other essential oils

Emotions Addressed: Stifled or blocked creativity, fear of self-expression, emotionally imbalanced, low will to live

Companion Oils: Tangerine, Wild Orange, Joyful Blend

Joyful Blend
The Oil of Joy

Joyful Blend was formulated as an antidepressant. This blend combines powerful mood stabilizers such as Sandalwood, Rose, Jasmine and Ylang Ylang with joy filled oils such as Tangerine, Elemi, Melissa and Lemon Myrtle. The warm vibrations of these and other oils used in Joyful Blend can soothe the heart and balance the emotions.

Joyful Blend can assist individuals in letting go of lower energy vibrations. Old habits and addictions lose their appeal as an individual shifts into higher levels of consciousness. This blend can raise one's energy levels and energetic vibrations into higher states. It can inspire feelings of cheerfulness, brightness, courage, relaxation, happiness, humor, playfulness and fun. By inspiring these feelings, Joyful Blend transforms depression into sunshine and joy. It teaches that worry and fear are not productive, but faith, hope and determination are. Joyful Blend powerfully persuades people to be happy, carefree and abundant. It supports individuals in flowing with life while remaining in peace and light.

Ingredients: Lavandin, Tangerine, Elemi, Lemon Myrtle, Melissa, Ylang Ylang and other essential oils

Emotions Addressed: Caught in low vibrations, depression, dark, serious, stern

Companion Oils: Tangerine, Melissa, Ylang Ylang, Wild Orange, Invigorating Blend

Massage Blend
The Oil of Relaxation

Massage Blend assists the body in calming, relaxing and releasing physical tension. On an emotional level, Massage Blend moves an individual from stiffness of heart and mind to openness and flexibility. This Blend is soothing to both body and mind and offers comfort in times of grief and sorrow.

Most people seek out massage when they are tense or stressed. Through bodywork and massage the individual is able to relax their tight muscles. Breathing may begin to regulate, slow and deepen. As an individual's body relaxes, so does their mind. As the muscles release tension, the heart can reopen to life. Circulation is enhanced, as is their ability to move with life and allow things to flow. This is the gift of the Massage Blend - the ability to relax, open and move in harmony once more with the body and with existence.

Ingredients: Basil, Grapefruit, Cypress, Marjoram and other essential oils

Emotions Addressed: Tense, stiffness in body or mind, stressed, unable to relax

Companion Oils: Tension Blend, Cypress, Basil, Peppermint, Calming Blend

Metabolic Blend
The Oil of Inner Beauty

In addition to supporting the physical aspects of weight loss, this blend may also be used to address the emotional patterns which underlie and contribute to one's weight. Individuals in need of the Metabolic Blend may set strict standards for themselves in diet or weight loss programs. They believe that by denying themselves of dietary pleasures and controlling their bodies they will force their desired result. Instead, their punitive withholding is met with whiplash from the body as it desperately seeks to survive. The need for foods and sweets becomes excessive, resulting in swings in diet, weight and mood. This usually causes discouragement and feeling out of control, as one berates themselves with criticism and self-hatred.

The Metabolic Blend can support individuals in releasing the heavy emotions which contribute to physical and emotional pounds. It encourages them to find feelings of self-worth. As they accept their body as it is, the body can more easily move towards its ideal expression. Metabolic Blend encourages individuals to rise above self-judgment by embracing the body's natural beauty and inherent value, regardless of weight, shape, or size.

Ingredients: Grapefruit, Lemon, Peppermint and other essential oils

Emotions Addressed: Self-criticism, worthlessness, feeling ugly, disgust or hate for physical appearance

Companion Oils: Grapefruit, Cinnamon, Patchouli, Focus Blend, Bergamot, Peppermint

Monthly Blend
The Oil of Vulnerability

Monthly Blend encourages warmth in relationships, stabilizes emotional imbalances and fosters emotional intimacy. It is a perfect blend for supporting pregnancy and child delivery, as it strengthens the mother-child bond. This blend assists women in accepting their maternal instincts and nurturing qualities.

Monthly Blend assists relationships by teaching individuals to be emotionally open and vulnerable. It eases the fear of rejection and encourages individuals to receive true warmth and love in their relationships. It also encourages feelings of empathy for others by reminding them to stay receptive to the thoughts, feelings and needs of other people.

This blend works as a powerful emotional stabilizer, especially during menstruation or menopause. It releases emotional tension within the reproductive organs and helps release the expectations of suffering and dread related to the monthly cycle. In short, Monthly Blend encourages emotional intimacy and assists individuals in emotional balancing.

Ingredients: Clary Sage, Lavender, Bergamot, Roman Chamomile, Cedarwood, Ylang Ylang, Geranium, Fennel, Carrot Seed and other essential oils

Emotions Addressed: Invulnerability, guarded, closed, dread of menstruation or menopause

Companion Oils: Myrrh, Women's Blend, Marjoram, Calming Blend, Geranium, Cedarwood, Ylang Ylang

Protective Blend
The Oil of Protection

This combination of oils is generally used to shield individuals from bacteria, mold and viruses. This blend's protective properties, however, extend beyond the physical level by aiding individuals in warding off energetic parasites, domineering personalities and other negative influences. The Protective Blend strengthens one's immune system, which governs the ability to defend against attacks from physical pathogens and negative energies.

Protective Blend is incredibly helpful for strengthening the inner Self along with the inner resolve to stand up for one's Self and live in integrity. This blend is especially indicated for personalities who have a weakened boundary due to some kind of perpetual violation to their personal space. Protective Blend gives individuals strength to say "no" and resolve to maintain clear boundaries. It cuts away unhealthy connections such as codependency, parasitic relationships or emotional viruses found in negative "group thought." Protective Blend greatly assists individuals in learning to stand up for themselves and live in integrity with their True Self.

Ingredients: Wild Orange, Clove, Cinnamon and other essential oils

Emotions Addressed: Attacked, unprotected, vulnerable, susceptibility to peer pressure

Companion Oils: Clove, Repellent Blend, Ginger

Repellent Blend
The Oil of Shielding

Repellent Blend was formulated as an insect repellent, but it also offers so much more. This blend helps individuals to stay calm in the face of danger or attack. Repellent Blend strengthens the protective shield around one's body, helping them to feel safe. This is especially important for children and adults who unconsciously "merge" with other people's energy. They may do this as a way to relieve others' burdens, or to simply "lighten the load" in the environment. Regardless of the motives, this type of energetic merging weakens an individual's energy system. Babies and young children are especially susceptible to trying to carry loved ones' feelings for them, as they struggle to know which emotions are theirs and which belong to other people. This blend can assist an individual in separating their own energy from another's.

While the confusion between boundaries is often unintentional, there are also those who would target or attack another person. Repellent Blend teaches individuals to hold strong boundaries and not allow themselves to be pushed around. It imbues individuals with courage and confidence to stand up for themselves and face their attackers.

Ingredients: Lemon Eucalyptus, Citronella and other essential oils

Emotions Addressed: Unprotected, attacked, defenseless, poor boundaries

Companion Oils: Melaleuca, Protective Blend, Clove, Ginger

Respiratory Blend
The Oil of Breath

Respiratory Blend addresses the inability to let go of grief and pain. The individual in need of Respiratory Blend struggles to breathe and literally feels suffocated by sadness. The lungs and air passages become constricted, preventing air and emotion from releasing. The root of this condition is feeling unloved; the individual grieves the love they never received. They often shut down due to fear, not knowing whether the love they need will be there. They distrust whether it's safe to open and take in life. Respiratory Blend encourages individuals to release grief and sadness, and to receive genuine love and healing.

Respiratory Blend also supports individuals' relationship with Spirit and deepens one's connection to life. It invites individuals to let go (breathe out) and receive (breathe in). In this way, this blend teaches individuals to embrace life through breath. Respiratory Blend imbues individuals with the courage to fully open.

Ingredients: Laurel Leaf (Bay), Peppermint, Eucalyptus, Melaleuca and other essential oils

Emotions Addressed: Sadness, grief, despair, unloved, difficulty breathing, constriction, distrust

Companion Oils: Lime, Eucalyptus, DNA Repairing Blend, White Fir, Calming Blend

Skin Clearing Blend
The Oil of Accepting Imperfections

Skin Clearing Blend was formulated for acne and general skin health. Its major ingredient, Black Cumin seed, is not an essential oil, but has trace amounts of essential oil within it. Black Cumin is prized in many Islamic countries for its healing properties. The Prophet Muhammad said, "In black cumin seed there is cure for every disease, except death." Skin Clearing Blend combines the healing properties of Black Cumin with other essential oils.

Skin Clearing Blend emotionally supports suppressed anger, guilt and self-judgment. The individual in need of this blend may harbor feelings of guilt or anger from the past. These deeply buried feelings may exist outside the individual's conscious awareness. Yet, these feelings of pain or anger literally "boil" to the surface. If the individual does not deal with these feelings appropriately, they may come out "sideways" through lashing out or blaming others.

Skin Clearing Blend supports individuals by increasing self-acceptance and self-love. It assists them in seeing their inherent worth, regardless of physical appearance. It encourages the healthy release and expression of feelings of anger. Skin Clearing Blend invites individuals to look past menial imperfections and to replace self-judgment with self-acceptance.

Ingredients: Black Cumin Seed, Ho Wood, Melaleuca, Litsea Berry and other essential oils

Emotions Addressed: Pain, anger, self-judgment

Companion Oils: Bergamot, Metabolic Blend, Melissa, Cinnamon

Soothing Blend
The Oil of Surrendering Pain

Soothing Blend is generally used for physical pain, but it can also assist individuals who are resisting or avoiding the emotions that *underlie* their physical pain. It gives a person strength to face their emotional wounds, allowing the wounds to surface for transformation and healing. This blend can teach individuals how to be the observer of their painful experiences rather than becoming over-identified with them. When a person suffers from intense emotional or physical pain, it is common for them to act irrationally or "lose their head." Soothing Blend can support the mind in staying cool and collected, regardless of the emotional turmoil or physical pain one may be in. In this way, the individual maintains mental clarity in the face of danger or pain.

At its core, Soothing Blend teaches individuals acceptance and tolerance of their pain. It reveals the possibility that pain is not cruel or bad, but is simply a teacher. Instead of resisting pain, one may embrace the lessons it has to offer. As one lets go of resistance, pain lessens and often dissipates altogether. By understanding the nature of pain, this blend encourages an assimilation of all life's experiences.

Ingredients: Wintergreen, Camphor, Peppermint, Blue Tansy, Blue Chamomile and other essential oils

Emotions Addressed: Resistance to pain, avoidance of emotional issues, hysteria in painful situations

Companion Oils: Anti-Aging Blend, Helichrysum, Wintergreen, Thyme

Tension Blend
The Oil of Relief

Formulated to relieve headaches, Tension Blend also assists individuals in releasing the stress and emotional tension that may have contributed to or caused their headache.

Tension Blend synergistically combines the powerful relaxation qualities of essential oils to assist and teach the body how to calm and relax. It can also help individuals release the fears that create tension and pain in the physical body. Tension Blend can calm severe stress, soothe trauma and bring balance to the body and energy system. This blend also helps in regaining equilibrium following periods of overwork, burnout and fatigue.

As physical and emotional discomforts are relieved, Tension Blend fosters feelings of appreciation. It reminds individuals to be grateful for and enjoy their many life experiences.

Ingredients: Wintergreen, Lavender, Peppermint, Frankincense, Cilantro, Roman Chamomile, Marjoram and other essential oils

Emotions Addressed: Stress, overworked, nervous, burnout, overwhelmed, fatigued

Companion Oils: Cypress, Massage Blend, Calming Blend, Soothing Blend

Women's Blend
The Oil of Femininity

The benefits of the Women's Blend are not limited to women alone. While this blend possesses a strong feminine quality, its female energy is often needed by both men and women.

Women's Blend softens the overly-masculine individual by getting them in touch with their feminine side. It encourages individuals to let go of pride and let down their tough exterior. When placed over the liver, Women's Blend can ease feelings of anger. It calms tension, irritability and malice, and encourages adaptability.

Women's Blend assists individuals in healing their relationships with their mothers, grandmothers and other women. It helps one reconnect with their mother when there has been strain, separation, loss, or abuse in the relationship. It challenges an individual to work through their issues relating to both femininity and sexuality. If one has rejected their feminine energy, this blend invites them to heal their wounds and find balance by reconnecting with their feminine side.

Ingredients: Patchouli, Bergamot, Sandalwood, Rose, Jasmine, Cinnamon, Cistus, Vetiver, Ylang Ylang and other essential oils

Emotions Addressed: Overly masculine, blocked or imbalanced female energy, unteachable, anger, irritable, tough exterior

Companion Oils: Monthly Blend, Myrrh, Geranium, Ylang Ylang, Bergamot

Section III

Appendices

Appendix A

Suggested Uses

Single Oils

Arborvitae: *The Oil of Divine Grace*

Aromatic: Inhale directly from the bottle at regular intervals throughout the day, or place a few drops into a diffuser.

Topical: Place 1-3 on the bottom of the feet and top of head, heart or chest. Dilute with carrier oil if desired.

Basil: *The Oil of Renewal*

Aromatic: Inhale directly from the bottle at regular intervals throughout the day, or place a few drops into a diffuser.

Topical: Place 3-5 drops over the adrenal glands or on the bottom of the feet in the morning and just before bed. Dilute with a carrier oil if desired.

Bergamot: *The Oil of Self-Acceptance*

Aromatic: Inhale directly from the bottle at regular intervals throughout the day, or place a few drops into a diffuser.

Topical: Place 2-3 drops over the solar plexus (upper stomach). Dilute with a carrier oil if desired.

Birch: *The Oil of Support*

Aromatic: Inhale directly from the bottle at regular intervals throughout the day, or place a few drops into a diffuser.

Topical: Place 1-3 drops along the spine or on the bottom of the feet. Dilute with a carrier oil if desired.

Massage: Dilute 2-3 drops with carrier oil and massage over the spine, back, or area of concern.

Black Pepper: *The Oil of Unmasking*

Aromatic: Inhale directly from the bottle at regular intervals throughout the day, or place a few drops into a diffuser.

Topical: Place 1-3 drops on the bottom of the feet. Dilute with a carrier oil if desired.

Cardamom: *The Oil of Objectivity*

Aromatic: Inhale directly from the bottle at regular intervals throughout the day, or place a few drops into a diffuser.

Topical: Place 1-3 over stomach, liver & gallbladder. Dilute with carrier oil if desired.

Cassia: *The Oil of Self Assurance*

Aromatic: Inhale directly from the bottle at regular intervals throughout the day, or place a few drops into a diffuser.

(Cassia continued)

Topical: Dilute one drop or less with carrier oil and place over the solar plexus (upper stomach).

Note: Cassia can be irritating to the skin; be cautious when using topically.

Cedarwood: *The Oil of Community*

Aromatic: Place 1-3 drops in the palm of hand, rub hands together and inhale.

Topical: Place one drop on forehead, or mix 3-4 drops with carrier oil and rub onto arms and the bottom of the feet.

Massage: Dilute 3-5 drops with carrier oil and massage onto feet or other chosen area.

Cilantro: *The Oil of Releasing Control*

Aromatic: Inhale directly from the bottle at regular intervals throughout the day, or place a few drops into a diffuser.

Topical: Place 1-3 drops over the stomach, liver, pancreas, along spine or on the bottom of the feet. Dilute with a carrier oil if desired.

Cinnamon: *The Oil of Sexual Harmony*

Aromatic: Inhale directly from the bottle at regular intervals throughout the day, or place a few drops into a diffuser.

(Cinnamon continued)

Topical: Dilute one drop with carrier oil and apply over pancreas.

Note: Cinnamon can be irritating to the skin; be cautious when using topically.

Clary Sage: *The Oil of Clarity & Vision*

Aromatic: Place 1-3 drops into a diffuser and place by bed at night. Also, inhale directly from the bottle regularly throughout the day.

Topical: Place 1-2 drops on the forehead or behind ears. Dilute with a carrier oil if desired.

Bath: Add 1-3 drops to bath just before for bed.

Massage: Place 3-5 drops on the bottom of the feet.

Clove: *The Oil of Boundaries*

Aromatic: Inhale directly from the bottle at regular intervals throughout the day, or place a few drops into a diffuser.

Topical: Place 2-3 drops on the bottom of the feet or over the stomach. Dilute with a carrier oil if desired.

Note: Clove can be irritating to the skin; be cautious when using topically.

Coriander: *The Oil of Loyalty*

Aromatic: Inhale directly from the bottle at regular intervals throughout the day, or place a few drops into a diffuser.

Topical: Place 1-3 drops over the solar plexus (upper stomach) and pancreas. Dilute with a carrier oil if desired.

Cypress: *The Oil of Motion & Flow*

Aromatic: Inhale directly from the bottle regularly throughout the day. Place 1-3 drops in the palm of the hand, rub hands together vigorously and inhale, or place a few drops into a diffuser.

Topical: Place 1-3 drops over the kidneys, just below the navel, or on the bottom of the feet. Dilute with a carrier oil if desired.

Bath: Add 1-3 drops to bath.

Massage: Dilute 3-5 drops with carrier oil and massage over entire body or other chosen area.

Eucalyptus: *The Oil of Wellness*

Aromatic: Place a large quantity of drops into a diffuser to disperse throughout the room or home environment.

Topical: Place 2-4 drops over the lungs, chest and throat. Dilute with a carrier oil if desired.

(Eucalyptus continued)

Bath: Add a drop in bath water when feeling ill.

Massage: Dilute 2-4 drops with carrier oil and massage over upper body.

Fennel: *The Oil of Responsibility*

Aromatic: Inhale directly from the bottle at regular intervals throughout the day, or place a few drops into a diffuser.

Topical: Place 1-3 drops over the stomach after meals or throughout the day. Dilute with a carrier oil if desired.

Massage: Dilute 1-2 drops with carrier oil and massage over abdomen.

Frankincense: *The Oil of Truth*

Aromatic: Inhale directly from the bottle at regular intervals throughout the day, or place a few drops into a diffuser.

Topical: Place 1-3 drops on the crown of the head, forehead, behind ears, or on the bottom of the feet. Dilute with a carrier oil if desired.

Bath: Add 1-3 drops to bath.

Mist: Place 3-10 drops into a spray bottle and mist around room, home, or other environment.

Massage: Dilute 3-5 drops with carrier oil and massage on skin.

Geranium: *The Oil of Love & Trust*

Aromatic: Inhale directly from the bottle at regular intervals throughout the day, or place a few drops into a diffuser.

Topical: Place 1-3 drops over the heart. Dilute with a carrier oil if desired.

Bath: Add 1-3 drops to bath.

Massage: Dilute 1-3 drops with carrier oil and massage over heart, chest, back, under arms or around lymph nodes.

Ginger: *The Oil of Empowerment*

Aromatic: Inhale directly from the bottle regularly throughout the day. Place a drop in the palm of the hand, rub hands together vigorously and inhale.

Topical: Place 1-3 drops over the stomach. Dilute with a carrier oil if desired.

Massage: Dilute 1-3 drops with carrier oil and massage over stomach, lower back or abdomen.

Grapefruit: *The Oil of Honoring the Body*

Aromatic: Inhale directly from the bottle at regular intervals throughout the day, or place a few drops into a diffuser.

(Grapefruit continued)

Topical: Place 1-3 drops on wrists, kidneys, liver or stomach. Dilute with a carrier oil if desired.

Massage: Dilute 1-3 drops with carrier oil and massage over kidneys or liver.

Helichrysum: *The Oil for Pain*

Aromatic: Inhale directly from the bottle at regular intervals throughout the day, or place a few drops into a diffuser.

Topical: Place 1-3 drops over the heart or on the spine. Dilute with a carrier oil if desired.

Bath: Add one drop to bath.

Massage: Dilute 1-3 drops with carrier oil and massage over spine and back or other chosen area.

Jasmine: *The Oil of Sexual Purity & Balance*

Aromatic: Inhale directly from the bottle at regular intervals throughout the day, wear as perfume, or place a few drops into a diffuser.

Topical: Place one drop on wrists, just below the naval, or wear as perfume. Dilute with carrier oil if desired.

Juniper Berry: *The Oil of Night*

Aromatic: Place a few drops into a diffuser just before bed and disperse throughout the bedroom.

Topical: Place a drop on the forehead or behind the ears before bed. Dilute with a carrier oil if desired.

Mist: Place 3-5 drops into a spray bottle and mist throughout bedroom just before bed.

Lavender: *The Oil of Communication*

Aromatic: Inhale directly from the bottle at regular intervals throughout the day, or place a few drops into a diffuser.

Topical: Place 1-3 drops over the throat, heart or solar plexus (upper stomach). Dilute with a carrier oil if desired.

Bath: Add 3-5 drops to bath.

Massage: Dilute 3-5 drops with carrier oil and massage over entire body or chosen area.

Lemon: *The Oil of Focus*

Aromatic: Inhale directly from the bottle at regular intervals throughout the day, or place a few drops into a diffuser.

Topical: Place 1-3 drops over the stomach or forehead. Dilute with a carrier oil if desired.

Lemongrass: *The Oil of Cleansing*

Aromatic: Inhale directly from the bottle at regular intervals throughout the day, or place a few drops into a diffuser.

(Lemongrass continued)

Topical: Place 1 drop on forehead, or 3-5 drops on the bottom of the feet, liver or kidneys. Dilute with a carrier oil if desired.

Mist: Place 10 drops in a spray bottle and mist around room, home or other environment.

Massage: Dilute 1-3 drops with carrier oil and massage on feet.

Note: Lemongrass can be irritating to the skin, be cautious when applying it topically.

Lime: *The Oil of Zest for Life*

Aromatic: Inhale directly from the bottle at regular intervals throughout the day, or place a few drops into a diffuser.

Topical: Place 1-3 drops over the lungs and chest. Dilute with a carrier oil if desired.

Marjoram: *The Oil of Connection*

Aromatic: Inhale directly from the bottle at regular intervals throughout the day, or place a few drops into a diffuser.

Topical: Place 1-3 drops over the heart. Dilute with a carrier oil if desired.

(Marjoram continued)

Massage: Dilute 3-5 drops with carrier oil and massage over sore muscles.

Melaleuca: *The Oil of Energetic Boundaries*

Aromatic: Inhale directly from the bottle at regular intervals throughout the day, or place a few drops into a diffuser.

Topical: Place 1-3 drops on the bottom of the feet. Dilute with a carrier oil if desired.

Mist: Place 3-5 drops into a spray bottle and mist around body.

Melissa: *The Oil of Light*

Aromatic: Inhale directly from the bottle at regular intervals throughout the day, or place a few drops into a diffuser.

Topical: Place one drop on forehead. Dilute with a carrier oil if desired.

Myrrh: *The Oil of Mother Earth*

Aromatic: Inhale directly from the bottle at regular intervals throughout the day, or place a few drops into a diffuser.

Topical: Place 1-3 drops over the heart, around the navel or on the bottom of feet. Dilute with a carrier oil if desired.

Oregano: *The Oil of Humility & Non-Attachment*

Aromatic: Inhale directly from the bottle at regular intervals throughout the day, or place a few drops into a diffuser.

Topical: Dilute one drop with carrier oil and rub on the bottom of the feet. Dilute with a carrier oil if desired.

Note: Oregano can be irritating to the skin; be cautious when applying topically.

Patchouli: *The Oil of Physicality*

Aromatic: Inhale directly from the bottle at regular intervals throughout the day, or place a few drops into a diffuser.

Topical: Place 1-3 drops on the bottom of the feet or just below the navel. Dilute with a carrier oil if desired.

Peppermint: *The Oil of a Buoyant Heart*

Aromatic: Place one drop in the palm of the hand, rub hands together vigorously and inhale. Or place a few drops into a diffuser.

Topical: Place 1-3 drops over the chest or stomach. Dilute with a carrier oil if desired.

Massage: Dilute 1-3 drops with carrier oil and massage over shoulders, head, neck or other chosen area.

Roman Chamomile: *The Oil of Spiritual Purpose*

Aromatic: Inhale directly from the bottle at regular intervals throughout the day, or place a few drops into a diffuser.

Topical: Place 3-6 drops over the stomach, or place one drop over forehead or behind the ears. Dilute with a carrier oil if desired.

Bath: Add 3-6 drops to bath.

Rose: *The Oil of Divine Love*

Aromatic: Inhale directly from the bottle regularly throughout the day.

Topical: Place one drop over the heart. Dilute with a carrier oil if desired.

Rosemary: *The Oil of Knowledge & Transition*

Aromatic: Inhale directly from the bottle at regular intervals throughout the day, or place a few drops into a diffuser.

Topical: Place 1-3 drops over the chest, neck, head and behind the ears. Dilute with a carrier oil if desired.

Sandalwood: *The Oil of Sacred Devotion*

Aromatic: Inhale directly from the bottle before meditating, studying or prayer.

Topical: Place one drop on the crown of the head or forehead. Dilute with a carrier oil if desired.

Tangerine: *The Oil of Cheer & Creativity*

Aromatic: Inhale directly from the bottle at regular intervals throughout the day, or place a few drops into a diffuser.

Topical: Place 1-2 drops on wrists, stomach, or heart. Dilute with a carrier oil if desired.

Thyme: *The Oil of Releasing & Forgiving*

Aromatic: Inhale directly from the bottle at regular intervals throughout the day, or place a few drops into a diffuser.

Topical: Dilute one drop with carrier oil and rub on the bottom of the feet.

Note: Thyme can be irritating to the skin; be cautious when applying topically.

Vetiver: *The Oil of Centering & Descent*

Aromatic: Inhale directly from the bottle regularly throughout the day, or place a drop in the palm of the hand, rub hands together vigorously and inhale.

(Vetiver continued)

Topical: Place 1-3 drops on the bottom of the feet. Dilute with a carrier oil if desired.

Massage: Dilute 1-3 drops with carrier oil and massage along spine and back.

White Fir: *The Oil of Generational Healing*

Aromatic: Inhale directly from the bottle at regular intervals throughout the day, or place a few drops into a diffuser.

Topical: Place 3-5 drops over lungs and chest or on the bottom of the feet. Dilute with a carrier oil if desired.

Bath: Add 1-3 drops to bath.

Massage: Dilute 1-3 drops with carrier oil and massage over chest, lungs, back, shoulders and around lymph nodes.

Wild Orange: *The Oil of Abundance*

Aromatic: Inhale directly from the bottle regularly throughout the day, or place a few drops into a diffuser and disperse at workplace.

Topical: Place 1-3 drops over the stomach or just below the navel. Dilute with a carrier oil if desired.

Bath: Add 1-3 drops to bath.

Wintergreen: *The Oil of Surrender*

Aromatic: Inhale directly from the bottle at regular intervals throughout the day, or place a few drops into a diffuser.

Topical: Place 2-3 drops over sore or tight muscles. Dilute with a carrier oil if desired.

Ylang Ylang: *The Oil of the Inner Child*

Aromatic: Inhale directly from the bottle at regular intervals throughout the day, or place a few drops into a diffuser.

Topical: Place 1-3 drops directly over the heart. Dilute with a carrier oil if desired.

Bath: Add 2-3 drops to bath.

Oil Blends

Anti-Aging Blend: *The Oil of Spiritual Insight*

Aromatic: Inhale directly from the bottle at regular intervals throughout the day, or place a small amount of oil in the palm of the hand, rub hands together vigorously and inhale.

Topical: Place a small amount of oil on the crown of the head, or roll over the forehead, behind ears, or on the bottom of the feet.

Calming Blend: *The Oil of Forgiveness*

Aromatic: Inhale directly from the bottle at regular intervals throughout the day, or place a few drops into a diffuser.

Topical: Place 1-3 drops over the heart or on the bottom of feet. Dilute with a carrier oil if desired.

Massage: Dilute with carrier oil and massage on feet or back.

Cleansing Blend: *The Oil of Purification*

Aromatic: Inhale directly from the bottle at regular intervals throughout the day, or place a few drops into a diffuser.

Topical: Place 1-3 drops over the liver, kidneys, along spine or on the bottom of the feet.

Mist: Place 10 or more drops into a spray bottle and mist around the home, environment or around body.

Detoxification Blend: *The Oil of Vitality & Transition*

Aromatic: Inhale directly from the bottle at regular intervals throughout the day, or place a few drops into a diffuser.

Topical: Place 3-5 drops over the liver or on the bottoms of feet. Dilute with a carrier oil if desired.

Massage: Dilute a few drops with carrier oil and massage along spine.

Digestive Blend: *The Oil of Digestion*

Aromatic: Inhale directly from the bottle at regular intervals throughout the day, or place a few drops into a diffuser.

Topical: Often work well applied over the stomach before or after meals, or throughout the day.

DNA Repairing Blend: *The Oil of Transformation*

Aromatic: Inhale directly from the bottle at regular intervals throughout the day, or place a few drops into a diffuser.

Topical: Place 3-5 drops along spine or on the bottom of the feet. Dilute with a carrier oil if desired.

Focus Blend: *The Oil of Presence*

Aromatic: Inhale directly from the bottle at regular intervals throughout the day, or place a small amount of oil in the palm of the hand, rub hands together vigorously and inhale.

(Focus Blend continued)

Topical: Roll oil onto the forehead, wrists and the bottom of the feet. Dilute with a carrier oil if desired.

Grounding Blend: *The Oil of Grounding*

Aromatic: Inhale directly from the bottle at regular intervals throughout the day, or place a few drops into a diffuser.

Topical: Place 3-5 drops along the spine or on the bottom of the feet. Dilute with a carrier oil if desired.

Invigorating Blend: *The Oil of Creativity*

Aromatic: Inhale directly from the bottle at regular intervals throughout the day, or place a few drops into a diffuser.

Topical: Place 1-3 drops over the stomach, liver, wrists or just below the navel. Dilute with a carrier oil if desired.

Joyful Blend: *The Oil of Joy*

Aromatic: Inhale directly from the bottle at regular intervals throughout the day, or place a few drops into a diffuser.

Topical: Place 1-3 drops on the forehead, behind ears, over stomach or on heart. Dilute with a carrier oil if desired.

Bath: Add 1-3 drops to bath.

Massage Blend: *The Oil of Relaxation*

Aromatic: Inhale directly from the bottle at regular intervals throughout the day, or place a few drops into a diffuser.

Massage: Dilute 3-5 drops with carrier oil and massage along shoulders, back, or other desired location.

Metabolic Blend: *The Oil of Inner Beauty*

Aromatic: Inhale directly from the bottle at regular intervals throughout the day, or place a few drops into a diffuser.

Topical: Place 1-3 drops over the stomach just before or after meals, or dilute with carrier oil and apply over hips, waist and body.

Monthly Blend: *The Oil of Vulnerability*

Aromatic: Inhale directly from the bottle at regular intervals throughout the day, or place a small amount of oil in the palm of the hand, rub hands together vigorously and inhale.

Topical: Rub oil onto hand and apply over the kidneys, liver, just below the navel, behind ears, or on the bottom of the feet. Dilute with a carrier oil if desired.

Protective Blend: *The Oil of Protection*

Aromatic: Inhale directly from the bottle at regular intervals throughout the day, or place a few drops into a diffuser.

(Protective Blend continued)

Topical: Place 3-5 drops on the bottom of the feet. Dilute with a carrier oil if desired.

Mist: Place 10 drops or more in a spray bottle and mist around body or room

Repellent Blend: *The Oil of Shielding*

Aromatic: Inhale directly from the bottle at regular intervals throughout the day, or place a few drops into a diffuser.

Topical: Place one drop in the palm of the hand, rub hands together vigorously and brush hands lightly over clothes and body or apply on wrists. Dilute with a carrier oil if desired.

Mist: Place 10 drops or more in a spray bottle and mist around body or room.

Respiratory Blend: *The Oil of Breath*

Aromatic: Inhale directly from the bottle at regular intervals throughout the day, or place a few drops into a diffuser. This oil works especially well being diffused in the environment.

Topical: Place 1-3 drops over the chest and lungs. Consider diluting with carrier oil to cover a larger area.

Skin Clearing Blend: *The Oil of Accepting Imperfections*

Aromatic: Inhale directly from the bottle at regular intervals throughout the day, or place a small amount of oil in the palm of the hand, rub hands together vigorously and inhale.

Topical: Rub oil onto face, neck, or other desired location. Dilute with a carrier oil if desired.

Soothing Blend: *The Oil of Surrendering Pain*

Aromatic: Inhale directly from the bottle at regular intervals throughout the day, or place a few drops into a diffuser.

Topical: Place 3-5 drops over shoulders, neck, back, or other area of pain and concern. Dilute with a carrier oil if desired.

Massage: Dilute a few drops with carrier oil and massage over area of concern.

Tension Blend: *The Oil of Relief*

Aromatic: Inhale directly from the bottle at regular intervals throughout the day, or place a small amount of oil in the palm of the hand, rub hands together vigorously and inhale.

Topical: Rub onto forehead, neck, behind ears or other areas of tension and concern.

Massage: Rub oil into the palm of your hand, dilute with a few drops of carrier oil and massage over area of tension or concern.

Women's Blend: *The Oil of Femininity*

Aromatic: Inhale directly from the bottle at regular intervals throughout the day, or place a few drops into a diffuser.

Topical: Place 1-3 drops just below the navel, over the heart, or on the bottom of the feet. Dilute with a carrier oil if desired.

Appendix B

Choosing and Applying Oils with Energy/Muscle Testing

Energy Testing

Energy testing, also known as muscle testing, is a quick and simple way to access information from a person's subconscious. The information is obtained by testing the energy of the body while asking a yes or no question. This testing allows us to bypass the conscious mind and tap into a deeper source of wisdom and knowledge. We recommend using energy testing to determine which oils you need, as well as how to apply them. In this book, when we suggest you "test" for something, we are referring to energy testing.

Choosing and Applying Oils

Choosing Which Oils to Use

The end of this appendix contains a list of single oils and a list of blends. These lists include all the oils discussed in this book. We have provided them as a convenient way for you to energy test which oils would be best for the situation you are trying to address.

The first step in choosing oils is to test to determine how many oils you need. Then, for each oil, test whether it is a single oil or a blend. You may want to phrase your testing like this: "The first most important oil I need is a single oil." "The second most important oil I need is a single oil" and so forth. A strong test indicates that yes, the oil is a single oil, while a weak test means no, it's not a single oil and therefore it must be a blend. Not only do these statements help you determine which types of oil you need, but they help you prioritize them from most important to least important.

Once you have determined how many oils you need and which are single and which are blends, use the appropriate list at the end of this appendix to test for the name of each oil.

How to Apply Oils

For a more complete description of how to apply essential oils see "How to Use Essential Oils" in Section I of this book.

For each oil you plan to use, test to determine the best method(s) for application:

1. Aromatic
2. Topical
3. Internal (See "A Word on Quality," in Section I)

Test for topical application, then test where to apply the oil:

Possible parts of the body for application

1. Arms
2. Back (upper/lower)
3. Brow/Forehead
4. Chest/Lungs
5. Crown
6. Ears
7. Face
8. Feet
9. Hands
10. Heart
11. Hips
12. Kidneys
13. Legs
14. Liver
15. Neck/Throat
16. Pancreas
17. Shoulders
18. Spine
19. Stomach
20. Toes
21. Waist

Amount and Frequency of Application

Once you know the method you will use to apply the oil, test for the following:

1. How many drops to use per application or how often to inhale from the bottle.
2. How many times per day to repeat the application, or, if you are using a diffuser, how many hours to diffuse the oil.
3. How many days to use the oil.

If testing reveals that you need to use more than one method of application for the same oil, repeat the steps above for each method.

Sample Testing Questions:

To test the number of drops:
"I need one drop of [name of oil]."
Then, "I need two drops of [name of oil]", etc.

To test how many times per day to apply the oil:
"I need [# drops you tested] drops once a day."
Then, "I need [# drops you tested] drops twice a day," etc.

To test how many days to take the oil:
"I need to take [name of oil] for one days"
Then, "I need to take [name of oil] for two days," etc.

Single Oils Testing List

1. Arborvitae
2. Basil
3. Bergamot
4. Birch
5. Black Pepper
6. Cardamom
7. Cassia
8. Cedarwood
9. Cilantro
10. Cinnamon
11. Clary Sage
12. Clove
13. Coriander
14. Cypress
15. Eucalyptus
16. Fennel
17. Frankincense
18. Geranium
19. Ginger
20. Grapefruit
21. Helichrysum
22. Jasmine
23. Juniper Berry
24. Lavender
25. Lemon
26. Lemongrass
27. Lime
28. Marjoram
29. Melaleuca
30. Melissa
31. Myrrh
32. Oregano
33. Patchouli
34. Peppermint
35. Roman Chamomile
36. Rose
37. Rosemary
38. Sandalwood
39. Tangerine
40. Thyme
41. Vetiver
42. White Fir
43. Wild Orange
44. Wintergreen
45. Ylang Ylang

Oil Blends Testing List

1. Anti-Aging Blend
2. Calming Blend
3. Cleansing Blend
4. Detoxification Blend
5. Digestive Blend
6. DNA Repairing Blend
7. Focus Blend
8. Grounding Blend
9. Invigorating Blend
10. Joyful Blend
11. Massage Blend
12. Metabolic Blend
13. Monthly Blend
14. Protective Blend
15. Repellent Blend
16. Respiratory Blend
17. Skin Clearing Blend
18. Soothing Blend
19. Tension Blend
20. Women's Blend

Appendix C

Essential Oil Emotional Usage Guide

A

Abandoned: Frankincense, Myrrh, Marjoram, Geranium

Abundance: Wild Orange, Invigorating Blend, Joyful Blend, Tangerine, Arborvitae

Abuse: Jasmine, Cinnamon, Clove, Helichrysum, White Fir, Cardamom

Accepted: Rose, Bergamot, Jasmine

Accountability: (see Responsibility)

Adaptable: Women's Blend

Addicted: Bergamot, Detoxification Blend, Frankincense, Jasmine, Peppermint, Vetiver, White Fir

Adjustment, difficulty with: Rosemary, Detoxification Blend

Afraid: (see Fear/Fearful)

Agitated: (see Irritated)

Alienated: Birch, Cedarwood, Myrrh, Arborvitae

Aloof: Marjoram, Grounding Blend, Jasmine, Detoxification Blend

Anger: Cardamom, Thyme, Calming Blend, Geranium, Ylang Ylang, Skin Clearing Blend, Women's Blend

Anguish: Helichrysum, Anti-Aging Blend, Melissa, Skin Clearing Blend

Annoyed: Rose, Cardamom, Calming Blend

Anxious/Anxiety: Basil, Respiratory Blend, Tension Blend

Apathy/Apathetic: Lemongrass, Vetiver, Lime, Detoxification Blend

Appearance, negative image of: (see Body, hate for)

Appetite, loss of: Digestive Blend, Fennel

Appreciative: (see Gratitude)

Apprehensive: Cassia, Cinnamon, Melissa

Approved of: Rose, Bergamot

Argumentative: Lavender, Cardamom

Arrogant: Women's Blend, Monthly Blend, Oregano

Ashamed: (see Shame)

Assertive: Clove, Black Pepper

Attacked: Protective Blend, Repellent Blend, Birch

Attached, overly: Oregano, Sandalwood, Detoxification Blend

Attentive: Lemon, Focus Blend

Authentic: Wild Orange, Cassia

Avoidance: Soothing Blend, Vetiver, Helichrysum, Grounding Blend, Juniper Berry, Jasmine

B

Barriers, emotional: Marjoram, Monthly Blend, Calming Blend, Rose

Beaten down: Protective Blend

Believing: (see Faith)

Belittled: Bergamot, Metabolic Blend

Bereaved: (see Grief)

Betrayed: Geranium, Rose, Ylang Ylang, Calming Blend

Bitterness: Calming Blend, Thyme

Blaming others: Cardamom, Skin Clearing Blend, Calming Blend, Vetiver, Ginger

Blaming self: Bergamot, Clove, Ginger

Blindness, spiritual: Anti-Aging Blend, Clary Sage, Lemongrass, Frankincense

Blocked, emotionally: Cypress, Thyme, Oregano

Body shame: Patchouli, Jasmine, Grapefruit, Metabolic Blend

Body tension: Tension Blend, Massage Blend, Patchouli

Body, disconnection from: Grounding Blend, Patchouli, Vetiver, Focus Blend, Jasmine

Body, hate for: Grapefruit, Metabolic Blend, Cinnamon, Skin Clearing Blend

Body, judgment of: Grapefruit, Metabolic Blend, Patchouli, Cinnamon, Skin Clearing Blend

Bonding: Geranium, Marjoram, Myrrh, Cedarwood

Boundaries, poor: Protective Blend, Melaleuca, Clove, Repellent Blend, Oregano, Cardamom

Bragging: (see Pride)

Brave: (see Courage)

Breath, constricted: Respiratory Blend, Massage Blend, Peppermint, White Fir, Arborvitae

Burdened: Anti-Aging Blend, White Fir, Wintergreen, Arborvitae, Tangerine, DNA Repairing Blend, Cilantro

Burned out: Basil, Tension Blend, Arborvitae, Respiratory Blend

C

Calm: Lavender, Lemon, Patchouli, Roman Chamomile, Sandalwood, Massage Blend, Calming Blend, Cardamom, Arborvitae, Women's Blend, Tension Blend, Focus Blend

Careless: (see Apathy/Apathetic)

Centered: Vetiver, Roman Chamomile, Clove, Cardamom

Change, resistance to: Cilantro,

Chaotic: Lemon, Vetiver, Cardamom

Cheated: (see Betrayed)

Cheerful: Tangerine, Lime, Wild Orange, Invigorating Blend, Joyful Blend, Arborvitae

Childish: Invigorating Blend

Clarity, mental: Lemon, Rosemary, Cardamom

Clarity, spiritual: Clary Sage, Frankincense, Sandalwood, Arborvitae, Lemongrass

Clean: Cleansing Blend, Lemongrass, Bergamot, Frankincense, Detoxification Blend, Jasmine

Clear-minded: Lemon, Cardamom

Clingy: Eucalyptus, Ylang Ylang

Closed, emotionally: Respiratory Blend, Ylang Ylang, Monthly Blend, Rose, Geranium, Jasmine, Detoxification Blend

Closed-minded: (see Narrow-minded)

Codependent: Melaleuca, Clove, Protective Blend, Cleansing Blend, Oregano, Ginger, Jasmine

Cold: (see Aloof)

Committed: Ginger, Coriander, Grounding Blend

Communication, blocked: Lavender, Monthly Blend

Compassion: Rose, Calming Blend, Geranium

Competitive: Women's Blend, Helichrysum, Arborvitae

Complaining: Joyful Blend, Ylang Ylang

Composed: Patchouli, Cardamom

Compulsive: Sandalwood, Black Pepper, Vetiver, Jasmine, Detoxification Blend

Conceited: Women's Blend, Oregano, Monthly Blend

Condemning: (see Judgmental)

Confidence: Bergamot, Cassia, Roman Chamomile, Lavender, Invigorating Blend

Conforming: Coriander, Clove, Ginger, Cassia

Confused/Confusion: Clary Sage, Lemon, Peppermint, Rosemary

Connected, emotionally: Marjoram, Vetiver, Cedarwood, Geranium

Connected, mentally: Rosemary, Cardamom, Lemon

Connected, physically: Patchouli, Grounding Blend

Connected, spiritually: Frankincense, Melissa, Roman Chamomile, Sandalwood

Consciousness, higher: Sandalwood, Anti-Aging Blend, Joyful Blend, Helichrysum, Frankincense

Constricted: Lavender, Cypress, Arborvitae, Detoxification Blend

Content: Tangerine, Arborvitae

Contentious: Cardamom, Calming Blend, Thyme

Controlled: Protective Blend, Clove, Coriander, Cilantro

Controlling: Cinnamon, Wintergreen, Cypress, Sandalwood, Metabolic Blend, Cilantro, Cardamom, Arborvitae

Courage: Helichrysum, Birch, Cassia, Clove, Ginger, Repellent Blend

Cowardly: (see Courage)

Cranky: Women's Blend, Calming Blend, Monthly Blend, Cardamom

Creative: Wild Orange, Tangerine, Invigorating Blend, Clary Sage

Creativity, blocked or stifled: Invigorating Blend, Tangerine, Wild Orange, Clary Sage

Crisis: Lavender, Basil, Peppermint, Geranium, Vetiver

Critical: Bergamot, Metabolic Blend, Thyme, Skin Clearing Blend, Cardamom

Cursed: Melissa

Cynical: Wild Orange, Tangerine, Skin Clearing Blend

D

Dark, fear of: Juniper Berry

Dark, in the: Anti-Aging Blend, Melissa, Clary Sage, Frankincense, Joyful Blend

Darkness: Lemongrass, Frankincense, Melaleuca, Anti-Aging Blend

Death wish: (see Suicidal)

Death, acceptance of: Roman Chamomile, Frankincense

Deceived: Clary Sage, Frankincense

Decisive: Lemon, Clove

Defeated: Clove, Invigorating Blend, Jasmine, Eucalyptus, Ginger, Fennel, Arborvitae

Defenseless: Repellent Blend, Protective Blend

Defensive: Oregano, Cardamom, Women's Blend, Monthly Blend, Ylang Ylang, Geranium

Defiant: Oregano, Cardamom, Women's Blend, Ylang Ylang

Defiled: Cleansing Blend, Thyme

Degraded: Bergamot, Clove

Denial: (see Avoidance)

Dependent: Melaleuca, Clove, Ginger, Jasmine

Depleted: Basil, Peppermint, Arborvitae, Jasmine

Depressed: Joyful Blend, Peppermint, Melissa

Desire, lack of: Grounding Blend, Fennel, Black Pepper, Jasmine, Invigorating Blend, Lemongrass, Detoxification Blend

Despair: Joyful Blend, Melissa, Bergamot, Respiratory Blend, Eucalyptus, Lemongrass, DNA Repairing Blend

Despondent: Lemongrass, Melissa, Detoxification Blend, Eucalyptus, Grounding Blend, Invigorating Blend

Dieting, addiction to: Bergamot, Detoxification Blend, Frankincense, Peppermint, Vetiver, White Fir

Discerning/Discernment: Clary Sage, Frankincense, Lemongrass

Disconnected from body: Patchouli, Grounding Blend, Focus Blend, Jasmine

Disconnection, spiritual: Frankincense, Sandalwood, Clary Sage

Discontent: Wild Orange, Cardamom, Skin Clearing Blend

Discouraged: Lime, Melissa, Joyful Blend, Wild Orange, Roman Chamomile, Anti-Aging Blend, DNA Repairing Blend

Disharmony: Grounding Blend, Calming Blend, Cardamom, Arborvitae

Disheartened: Rose, Geranium

Dishonest: Black Pepper, Vetiver, Cassia, Lavender, Geranium, Monthly Blend

Distant: Marjoram, Jasmine, Cedarwood, Arborvitae

Distracted: Focus Blend

Distraught: Anti-Aging Blend, Lemongrass

Distrusting: Geranium, Marjoram, Myrrh, Arborvitae, Jasmine

Divided/Double minded: Grounding Blend, Vetiver, Lemon

Dominated: Clove, Protective Blend, Repellent Blend, Ginger

Doubtful: Sandalwood, DNA Repairing Blend

Drained: Basil, Melaleuca, Tension Blend, Massage Blend, Arborvitae

Dread: Fennel, Monthly Blend

Drudgery: Roman Chamomile, Coriander, Invigorating Blend, Fennel

Dull: Invigorating Blend, Wild Orange, Roman Chamomile, Detoxification Blend

Dumb, feeling: Lemon, Peppermint, Rosemary

E

Egotistical: Women's Blend, Oregano, Arborvitae, Rose

Elevated: Joyful Blend, Lime, Melissa

Embarrassed: Cassia, Jasmine

Empathy: Monthly Blend, Geranium, Rose

Empowered: Arborvitae, Ginger, Clove

Emptiness: Vetiver, Sandalwood, Arborvitae

Energized: Basil, Respiratory Blend, Arborvitae

Energy, lack of: Lemon, Peppermint, Wild Orange, Arborvitae, Joyful Blend, Invigorating Blend

Enlightened: Melissa, Frankincense, Sandalwood

Entangled: Melaleuca, Clove, Protective Blend, Oregano

Enthusiasm: Melissa, Respiratory Blend

Envy: (See Jealousy)

Escapism: Vetiver, Focus Blend, Patchouli, Grounding Blend, Jasmine

Estranged: (see Separated)

Exasperated: Basil, Respiratory Blend, Lavender

Excessive: Grounding Blend, Sandalwood, Jasmine

Exhausted: Basil

F

Façade, emotional: Black Pepper, Vetiver, Soothing Blend, Helichrysum

Failure, feeling like: Bergamot, Roman Chamomile

Faith: Anti-Aging Blend, Sandalwood, Arborvitae

Faithless: Anti-Aging Blend, Sandalwood, Arborvitae

Father, issues with: Frankincense

Fatigue, mental: Lemon, Respiratory Blend, Rosemary

Fatigued: Basil, Respiratory Blend, Tension Blend

Fear/Fearful: Juniper Berry, Cassia, Cinnamon, Jasmine, Birch, Cypress, Lavender, Myrrh, Arborvitae

Fearless: Juniper Berry, Clove

Firm: Clove, Birch

Flexibility: Cypress, Massage Blend, Arborvitae, Wild Orange

Flighty: Grounding Blend

Focus, inability to: Lemon, Peppermint

Focused: Lemon, Rosemary, Grounding Blend, Cardamom, Roman Chamomile

Food, addiction to: Grapefruit, Metabolic Blend, Detoxification Blend

Foolish, feeling: Cassia

Forgetful: Lemon, Peppermint

Forgiveness: Geranium, Thyme, Calming Blend

Fragmented: Vetiver, Cardamom, Grounding Blend

Frantic: (see Hurried)

Friendless: Marjoram, Cedarwood

Frustrated: Geranium, Cardamom, Roman Chamomile

Fulfilled: Roman Chamomile, Jasmine

G

Generational issues: White Fir, DNA Repairing Blend, Birch, Jasmine

Gentle: Geranium, Ylang Ylang, Anti-Aging Blend

Giving up: Helichrysum, Soothing Blend, Detoxification Blend

Gratitude: Wild Orange, Helichrysum, Tension Blend, Anti-Aging Blend

Greedy: Wild Orange

Grief: Respiratory Blend, Soothing Blend, Geranium, Lime

Grouchy: Cardamom, Women's Blend, Thyme

Grounded: Grounding Blend, Birch, Patchouli, Vetiver, Focus Blend, Arborvitae, Anti-Aging Blend

Guarded: Monthly Blend, Jasmine

Guilt: Bergamot, Lemon, Peppermint, Skin Clearing Blend

H

Harassed: Protective Blend, Repellent Blend

Hardened: Rose, Geranium, Calming Blend, Ylang Ylang, Jasmine, Tangerine

Hard-hearted: Rose, Geranium, Calming Blend, Thyme

Harsh: Cardamom, Marjoram, Geranium

Hate/Hatred: Thyme, Cardamom

Haughty: (see Egotistical)

Haunted: Frankincense, Protective Blend, Melissa

Headstrong: Cardamom, Oregano, Wild Orange, Women's Blend, Lime

Healed: Helichrysum, Geranium, Eucalyptus, Jasmine

Heartbroken: Geranium, Rose

Heartless: Rose, Geranium, Cardamom

Heavy-hearted: Lime, Calming Blend, Joyful Blend, Geranium

Helpless/Helplessness: Clove, Ginger, Protective Blend

Hereditary issues: (see Generational Issues)

Hesitant: (see Indecisive)

Hiding: Cassia, Black Pepper

High-strung: Massage Blend

Hoarding: Lemongrass, Myrrh, Cleansing Blend, Detoxification Blend, Thyme, Wild Orange

Holding back: Cassia, Lavender, Jasmine

Holding onto the past: Thyme, Lemongrass, Cleansing Blend, Detoxification Blend, Wintergreen

Honest: Black Pepper, Geranium, Lavender

Hopeless: Melissa, Clary Sage, Anti-Aging Blend

Humiliated: Cassia

Humor, sense of: Wild Orange, Joyful Blend

Hurried: Massage Blend, Tension Blend

Hurtful to others: Cardamom, Women's Blend, Calming Blend, Rose

Hypocritical: Clary Sage, Frankincense

Hysterical: Grounding Blend, Soothing Blend

I

Illness, attached to: Eucalyptus

Imbalanced, emotionally: Calming Blend, Invigorating Blend

Immature, emotionally: Geranium, Fennel

Immobilized: Cypress, Thyme

Immoral: Frankincense, Detoxification Blend, Cleansing Blend, Jasmine, Vetiver

Impatient/Impatience: (see Anxiety)

Impoverished: Wild Orange

Imprisoned: Eucalyptus, Lavender, Detoxification Blend

Inadequate: Bergamot, Metabolic Blend, Skin Clearing Blend

Incapable: Bergamot

Inconsiderate of others: Cardamom, Cinnamon, Calming Blend

Inconsistent: Grounding Blend, Coriander

Indecisive: Lemon, Peppermint

Indifferent: (see Apathy/Apathetic)

Inferior: Bergamot

Inflexible: Cypress, Massage Blend, Arborvitae, Wild Orange

Innocent: Ylang Ylang, Geranium, Jasmine

Insecure: Cassia, Bergamot

Insignificant: Roman Chamomile

Instability: Grounding Blend, Arborvitae

Intimidated: Clove, Repellent Blend, Ginger

Intolerant: Geranium, Cardamom, Rose, Skin Clearing Blend

Introvert: Marjoram, Cedarwood

Invigorated: Peppermint, Lemon, Invigorating Blend

Invulnerable: Monthly Blend, Marjoram

Irresponsible: Fennel, Ginger, Grounding Blend

Irritated: Women's Blend, Calming Blend, Monthly Blend, Cardamom

Isolated: Cedarwood, Arborvitae, Marjoram

J

Jealousy: Cinnamon, Calming Blend

Joy, lack of: Joyful Blend, Arborvitae, Lemon, Ylang Ylang

Joyful: Lemon, Lime, Wild Orange, Tangerine, Peppermint, Ylang Ylang, Invigorating Blend, Joyful Blend, Arborvitae

Judged: Birch, Clove, Ginger, Cassia

Judgmental: Cardamom, Women's Blend, Calming Blend, Geranium, Rose, Ylang Ylang, Black Pepper

K

Kindness: Anti-Aging Blend, Geranium

Know-it-all: Oregano, Women's Blend, Rosemary, Wintergreen, Sandalwood

L

Learning Disorders: Lemon, Rosemary, Digestive Blend

Left out: Cedarwood, Marjoram, Myrrh

Lethargy: Lemongrass, Invigorating Blend

Liberated: Detoxification Blend, Cleansing Blend, Lavender, Melissa, Arborvitae

Light-hearted: (see Joyful)

Limited thinking: Oregano, Rosemary, Coriander, Digestive Blend

Loneliness: Marjoram, Cedarwood, Frankincense, Myrrh

Loss: Geranium, Ylang Ylang

Lost/Purposeless: Roman Chamomile, Frankincense

Love, unconditional: Rose, Geranium, Calming Blend

Loved: Frankincense, Rose, Respiratory Blend

Low self-esteem/Self-worth: Bergamot, Metabolic Blend, Jasmine, Skin Clearing Blend

Loyal: Coriander, Jasmine

Lustful: Cinnamon, Jasmine

M

Mad: (see Anger)

Manipulated: Clove, Protective Blend

Manipulative: Cinnamon, Monthly Blend

Masculine, overly: Women's Blend, Monthly Blend

Masking, emotional: Black Pepper

Materialistic: Sandalwood, Oregano, Cilantro, Detoxification Blend

Maternal connection, disrupted: Myrrh, Monthly Blend, Women's Blend

Mature, emotionally: Geranium, Fennel

Mean: Geranium, Ylang Ylang, Cardamom, Women's Blend, Monthly Blend

Melancholy: (see Sadness, Depressed)

Menopause, dread of: Monthly Blend, Jasmine, Grapefruit

Menstruation, dread of: Monthly Blend, Jasmine, Grapefruit

Moody/Unstable moods: Joyful Blend

Motivated: Invigorating Blend, Black Pepper

Moving forward: (see Stagnant)

N

Narrow-minded: Rosemary, Oregano, Wild Orange, Lemon

Need for approval: Bergamot

Neglected: Monthly Blend, Cedarwood, Myrrh, Marjoram

Nervousness: Basil, Wild Orange, Tension Blend

Nightmares: Juniper Berry

Not enough: (see Scarcity)

O

Obsessed: Patchouli, Jasmine, Grounding Blend, Detoxification Blend

Obsessive-compulsive: Bergamot, Sandalwood, Cleansing Blend, Jasmine

Offended: Calming Blend, Geranium

Open-minded: Clary Sage, Wild Orange, Massage Blend

Opinionated: Oregano

Oppressed: Clove, Protective Blend, White Fir

Optimism: Melissa, Invigorating Blend, Tangerine, Bergamot

Out of control: Cardamom, Grounding Blend, Jasmine

Over-analyzing: Wild Orange, Ylang Ylang

Overly-empathetic: (see Boundaries, poor)

Overstimulation: Digestive Blend, Grounding Blend

Overthinking: Sandalwood, Myrrh, Ylang Ylang, Wild Orange

Overwhelmed: Basil, Massage Blend, Tension Blend, Digestive Blend, Tangerine

Overworked: Wild Orange, Ylang Ylang, Tension Blend, Arborvitae, Tangerine

P

Pain, emotional: Helichrysum, Soothing Blend, Geranium, Skin Clearing Blend

Pain, resistance to: Soothing Blend, Helichrysum

Panic: Grounding Blend, Soothing Blend

Patience: Cardamom, Grounding Blend, Anti-Aging Blend

Peaceful: Roman Chamomile, Joyful Blend, Cardamom, Arborvitae

Peer pressure: Ginger, Clove, Protective Blend

Perfectionism: Cypress, Arborvitae, Calming Blend, Cardamom

Persecuted: Protective Blend

Perseverance: Helichrysum, Grounding Blend

Pessimistic: Wild Orange, Peppermint

Poor, financially: Wild Orange

Possessive: Sandalwood, Oregano, Wintergreen

Powerless to heal: Arborvitae, Eucalyptus

Powerless: Clove, Ginger, Arborvitae, Jasmine

Pretense: Black Pepper, Cinnamon

Pride: Oregano, Women's Blend, Sandalwood, Wintergreen

Procrastination: Focus Blend

Protected: Protective Blend, Clove, Repellent Blend, Frankincense, Juniper Berry

Punishing, self: Bergamot, Jasmine, Metabolic Blend

Pure: Jasmine, Cleansing Blend, Lemongrass

Purposeful: Roman Chamomile, Ginger

Purposeless: Roman Chamomile

Q

Quarrelsome: Women's Blend, Oregano, Cardamom

Quick-tempered: Cardamom, Geranium, Monthly Blend

Quitting: Helichrysum, Arborvitae

R

Rage: Cardamom, Thyme

Rational: Lemon, Cardamom

Reclusive: Marjoram, Cedarwood

Reinforced: Protective Blend, Birch, Cedarwood, Arborvitae

Rejection, fear of: Lavender, Cinnamon, Lime

Relationships, codependent: Melaleuca, Clove, Protective Blend, Ginger, Jasmine

Relationships, parasitic: Melaleuca, Protective Blend, Oregano, Jasmine, Detoxification Blend

Relaxed: Tension Blend, Calming Blend, Arborvitae, Lavender, Roman Chamomile

Relieved: Helichrysum, Tension Blend, Arborvitae, Peppermint

Renewed: Basil, Peppermint, Arborvitae

Repressed: Lavender, Vetiver, Black Pepper, Jasmine

Resentment: Calming Blend, Geranium, Thyme, Cardamom

Resignation: Lime, Melissa, Detoxification Blend

Resistance: Arborvitae, Vetiver, Soothing Blend, Digestive Blend

Resolute: Birch

Responsibility: Ginger, Fennel, Cardamom, Grounding Blend

Revitalized: Basil, Respiratory Blend, Lime, Detoxification Blend

Rigid: Cypress, Arborvitae, Oregano, Wild Orange, Tangerine

Rushed: (see Hurried)

S

Sadness: Respiratory Blend, Calming Blend, Ylang Ylang, Geranium, Peppermint, Massage Blend

Scarcity: Wild Orange, Arborvitae

Scattered: Vetiver, Grounding Blend, Focus Blend

Secure: (see Protected)

Self, weak sense of: Lemon, Bergamot, Vetiver, Ginger, Jasmine, Grounding Blend, Fennel

Self-acceptance: Bergamot, Grapefruit, Metabolic Blend, Jasmine, Lemon

Self-assured: (see Confidence)

Self-betrayal: Coriander

Self-criticism: Metabolic Blend, Bergamot

Self-doubt: (see Confidence)

Self-expression: Lavender, Invigorating Blend, Jasmine

Self-judgment: Bergamot, Metabolic Blend

Self-love: (see Self-Acceptance)

Self-sabotage: Metabolic Blend

Sensitive, overly: Repellent Blend, Protective Blend, Clove, Ginger

Separated: Myrrh, Frankincense, Cedarwood, Arborvitae

Serious, overly: Tangerine, Invigorating Blend, Joyful Blend, Wild Orange

Sexual identity, acceptance of: Cinnamon, Jasmine

Sexual repression: Jasmine, Cinnamon

Sexually imbalanced: Jasmine, Cinnamon, Women's Blend

Shame, body: Patchouli, Grapefruit, Metabolic Blend, Jasmine

Shame: Bergamot, Frankincense

Shock: Lavender, Basil, Peppermint, Wintergreen

Shy: Cassia, Cinnamon, Ginger

Sickly: Eucalyptus, Patchouli

Soothed: Soothing Blend, Massage Blend, Tension Blend, Joyful Blend

Soul, dark night of: Anti-Aging Blend, Melissa, Frankincense, Helichrysum

Speaking, fear of: Lavender, Jasmine

Spontaneity: Wild Orange, Invigorating Blend, Tangerine

Stable: Grounding Blend

Stagnant: (see Stuck)

Stern: Joyful Blend, Wild Orange, Invigorating Blend, Women's Blend

Stiffness (body or mind): Massage Blend, Cypress

Strength: Birch, Protective Blend, Wintergreen, Arborvitae

Stressed: Massage Blend, Calming Blend, Ylang Ylang, Tension Blend, Basil

Stubborn: Wintergreen, Oregano, Arborvitae

Stuck: Cypress, Lemongrass, Thyme, Detoxification Blend, Birch, Fennel, DNA Repairing Blend

Suicidal: Invigorating Blend, Melissa, Anti-Aging Blend, Frankincense, Lime

Superficial: Black Pepper

Supported: Birch, Cedarwood, Arborvitae

Surrender: Wintergreen, Arborvitae, Sandalwood

T

Teachable: Wintergreen, Oregano, Rosemary

Tenderhearted: Geranium, Calming Blend, Rose, Ylang Ylang

Tense: Massage Blend, Tension Blend, Cypress, Arborvitae, Women's Blend

Terror/Terrified: Juniper Berry

Thankful: (see Gratitude)

Timid: (see Shy)

Tired: Basil, Invigorating Blend, Detoxification Blend

Tolerant: Thyme, Cardamom, Geranium, Soothing Blend

Toxic energy: Lemongrass, Melaleuca, Cardamom, Detoxification Blend, Cleansing Blend

Toxicity: Melaleuca, Detoxification Blend, Cleansing Blend, Detoxification Blend, Lemongrass, DNA Repairing Blend, Cilantro

Transitioning, difficulty with: Rosemary, Detoxification Blend, DNA Repairing Blend

Trapped: Lavender, Thyme, Cleansing Blend, Detoxification Blend, Black Pepper, Cilantro, Arborvitae, Jasmine

Trauma, Emotional: Geranium, Calming Blend, Clove, Helichrysum, Jasmine, Ylang Ylang

Trust: Geranium, Marjoram, Myrrh, Rosemary, Jasmine, Anti-Aging Blend

U

Ugly, feeling: Metabolic Blend, Grapefruit, Skin Clearing Blend

Undecided: (see Indecisive)

Unforgiving: Thyme, Calming Blend, Rose, Geranium, Cardamom

Unfulfilled: Jasmine, Roman Chamomile

Ungrateful: (see Gratitude)

Ungrounded: Grounding Blend, Focus Blend, Vetiver, Patchouli, Myrrh, Birch, Arborvitae

Unheard: Lavender

Unlovable: Bergamot, Respiratory Blend, Jasmine

Unloving: Geranium, Rose, Cardamom, Calming Blend, Thyme

Unprotected: Protective Blend, Repellent Blend

Unsafe in the world: Myrrh, Protective Blend, Jasmine

Unseen: Lavender, Cassia

Unsettled: Roman Chamomile, Cardamom

Unsupported: Birch, Cedarwood, Arborvitae

Unteachable: Rosemary, Women's Blend, Oregano

Unyielding: (see Stubborn)

Upheld: (see Supported)

V

Victim: Clove, Ginger, Jasmine, Skin Clearing Blend

Violated: Protective Blend, Ginger, Clove, Jasmine

Violent: Cardamom, Calming Blend, Frankincense

Virtuous: Jasmine, Cinnamon, Frankincense

Vision, spiritual: Clary Sage

Vulnerable: Monthly Blend, Jasmine, Protective Blend, Arborvitae, Repellent Blend

W

Weak-willed: Birch, Melaleuca, Ginger, Clove, Wintergreen

Whole-minded: Rosemary

Willful, excessively: Oregano, Wintergreen, Cardamom, Arborvitae

Withdrawn: (see Isolated)

Workaholic: Wild Orange, Ylang Ylang, Tangerine, Arborvitae, Invigorating Blend

Worried: Wild Orange, Tangerine, Sandalwood, Cilantro

Worthless, feeling: Cassia, Bergamot, Metabolic Blend

Wounded: Helichrysum, Jasmine

Appendix D

How to Host a Class on Emotions & Essential Oils

General Guidelines

In this appendix we suggest classes you may host on *Emotions & Essential Oils*. Note that the following class suggestions utilize this book's companion audio lecture, a CD entitled, *Emotions & Essential Oils: The Five Stages of Healing*. This audio lecture is available at www.enlightenhealing.com/deo/.

Keep in mind that the individual hosting these classes should ideally have an ample amount of experience with emotional healing themselves. To direct a class, and assist others in keeping their comments appropriate, it is best to have some experience in this area. This does not mean you have to be an emotional health expert, just that you have some experience with the subject.

Note: It is always a good practice following any class to encourage the group to practice the material presented, by using the essential oils and free writing regularly. If your group is unfamiliar with free writing, you may want to briefly explain the process or simply play the bonus track from the audio lecture mentioned above (track 10) for the group.

Class Option A: Introductory Class

Class Option A introduces the concept of emotional healing with essential oils - that it's possible! This class is ideal for those that are new or unfamiliar with the concept.

Steps:

1) Introduce this book, *Emotions & Essential Oils* to the class. Explore its basic premise: that in addition to their physical properties, essential oils assist in emotional healing as well.

   Consider summarizing concepts from the audio lecture *Emotions & Essential Oils: The Five Stages of Healing* or from this book to share with the class. If you are uncomfortable sharing in front of a group, or do not feel you understand the material adequately enough to share with others, consider sharing track 2 or 3 from the audio lecture, *Emotions & Essential Oils: The Five Stages of Healing* and discussing it with the group. Or you may want to read "Healing Emotions with Essential Oils" from Section I of this book, pages 7-10. If you share from the audio lecture or this book, take a few minutes to discuss what you share with the group and answer any questions.

2) Share appropriate personal experiences and stories you have encountered about the emotional healing properties of oils. Keep this section brief and to the point. If you do not have any stories or personal experiences to share with the group, consider reading "Kallie's Story" from Section I of this book.

Note: Do not try to convince your audience that oils work on this level. Each person must come to an understanding of oils' subtle healing abilities on their own. While offering a small amount of scientific background or evidence on the subject may be helpful for your audience, trying to convince or persuade individuals will never work. Allow people space and room to grow, in their own way, and in their own timing. Do not give them more information than they are ready for, or more than they can handle at one time. You must be sensitive to the needs, and maturity level of the specific group you are working with. Most individuals need some time (months to years) to work with essential oils on the physical level before they are ready or even willing to explore the subtle nature of the oils.

3) Choose either activity one or two from the audio lecture, *Emotions & Essential Oils: The Five Stages of Healing* to do with the group. You may either summarize these activities in your own words, or play the tracks from the audio CD for the group.

   Activity One
   - Track 4 Stage Two: Healing the Heart (this track establishes a foundation for the first activity)
   - Track 5 Activity One
   - Track 6 Invitation & Clarifications for Activity One

   Activity Two
   - Track 7 Activity Two
   - Track 8 Invitation & Clarifications for Activity Two

4) Invite the class to experiment with the emotional properties of essential oils. Challenge them to regularly use the oil(s) they chose from the activity.

5) Wrap up the class. If you feel comfortable answering people's questions, take a few moments to do so.

Class Option B: Intermediate Class

Class Option B highlights one essential oil, exploring it in detail. The purpose of this class is to allow the presenter an opportunity to study an essential oil in depth and practice sharing in front of a group. This class can also provide a deeper understanding of the oils for those attending. The aim of the class is to explore the physical and the emotional properties of an essential oil. Keep in mind the preparation for such a class may be extensive.

Steps:
1) Just as before, take a moment to introduce this book, *Emotions & Essential Oils*, and discuss its basic premise: that in addition to their physical properties, essential oils assist in emotional healing as well. Explain that you will be discussing *both* the physical and emotional properties of an essential oil at length.

2) Introduce the essential oil that you have chosen to highlight. You may want to discuss the reasons why you chose this specific essential oil to research and share for the class.

Consider discussing the essential oil's:
- History, Name (meaning of)
- Plant type/species
- Which part of the plant is used/distilled
- The region of the world the plant is grown
- Odor, intensity, what oils it blends well with
- Chemical constituents
- **Common physical uses**
- **Emotional properties of the oil**

As you discuss the physical properties of the oil you may want to share scientific research or other studies you have gathered on that essential oil. As you explore the emotional properties of the oil, consider sharing personal experiences or other healing stories you have encountered in relation to that specific essential oil. Again, do not try to convince your audience that oils work on the emotional level. While offering a small amount of scientific background or evidence on the subject may be helpful to your audience, trying to convince or persuade individuals will never work. Be sensitive to the needs and maturity level of the specific group you are working with.

3) Consider creating interactive games or other activities to assist the learning of the group. You may want to use activities one or two from the audio lecture, *Emotions & Essential Oils: The Five Stages of Healing* (see Class Option A for more instructions on using this lecture in a class). Or create games and activities of your own.

4) You may want to offer practical suggestions on how to use the essential oil you have discussed. Also invite the class to apply the information by using the essential oil regularly and engaging with the oils through free writing (see the bonus track, track 10 from the audio lecture, *Emotions & Essential Oils: The Five Stages of Healing*).

5) Wrap up the class. If you feel comfortable answering people's questions, take a few moments to do so.

Important Disclaimer:

These classes are for educational purposes only. None of the information contained in this section can or should be used as a means for prescribing or diagnosing another individual. There is no permission given or implied to practice counseling or therapy without a license. Those with psychological or emotional disorders should consult with a licensed health care professional for appropriate treatment. These classes should never be used as a substitute for professional counseling, support groups, or addiction recovery programs.

How to Order Books

Purchasing Additional Materials

To order *Emotions & Essential Oils* and other helpful products visit:

www.enlightenhealing.com/deo/

Purchasing Books in Bulk

If you would like to share this book with others, we have prepared reduced pricing for those interested in buying in bulk. Bulk pricing is found on the product pages of our website.